REPRODUCTIVE HEALTH AWARENESS
Among the Tribal Women in Manipur

About the Author

Rose Nembiakkim did her post-graduation in Social Work from the University of Delhi and M.Phil from the Centre for Social Medicine and Community Health, Jawaharlal Nehru University, New Delhi. Presently, she is a lecturer in Staff Training and Research Institute of Distance Education (STRIDE), Indira Gandhi National Open University.

Earlier, Rose Nembiakkim was a lecturer in Social Work at the University of Delhi. She has also worked as a Project Officer with Sangini (India) Trust. She has co-edited a book, titled *Legal Rights of Sexual Minority*, published by the Sangini (India) Trust.

REPRODUCTIVE HEALTH AWARENESS

AMONG THE TRIBAL WOMEN IN MANIPUR

Rose Nembiakkim

CONCEPT PUBLISHING COMPANY, NEW DELHI-110059

Cataloging in Publication Data—DK
Courtesy: D.K. Agencies (P) Ltd. <docinfo@dkagencies.com>

Nembiakkim, Rose.
Reproductive health awareness : among the tribal women in Manipur / Rose Nembiakkim.
p. cm.
With special reference to Churachandpur District of Manipur, India.
Includes bibliographical references (p.)
Includes index.
ISBN 13: 9788180695094
ISBN 10: 8180695093

1. Reproductive health—India—Churachandpur (District). 2. Tribes—Health and hygiene—India—Churachandpur (District). 3. Poor women—Health and hygiene—India—Churachandpur (District). 4. Church work with women—India—Churachandpur (District). I. Title.

ISBN-13: 978-81-8069-509-4
ISBN-10: 81-8069-509-3

First Published 2008

Published and Printed by
Ashok Kumar Mittal
Concept Publishing Company
A/15-16, Commercial Block, Mohan Garden
New Delhi (INDIA)

Phones : 25351460, 25351794
Fax : 091-11-25357103
Email : publishing@conceptpub.com

Acknowledgements

First and foremost I would like to thank God for giving me the good health to finish my present work.

I would like to express my gratitude to my father (Late) Thangkhanpau Guite, who taught me the meaning of education and because of whom I am able to write this book. My sincere gratitude to my mother Mrs. Pauneihoi Guite, who stoically believed in me so that the lessons taught by my father do not go in vain.

I am grateful to my sisters Grace, Mercy and Niang and to my brother John who understood my objectives and gave me unflinching support.

I am thankful to my Supervisor Dr. Sanghmitra Acharya for her valuable suggestions and active cooperation in the selection of topic of the present work and her expert guidance during initial phase of the study particularly to prepare research protocol and preparing the research tools. I thank her for believing in my potential.

I would like to express my sincere thanks to Mr. Jelkhanthang and family, who helped me with my fieldwork and made available to me the important literature regarding Manipur State.

I would like to make use of this opportunity to thank my friends and well-wishers without whose valuable comments and suggestion this dissertation could not be produced in the present form.

My acknowledgement would not be complete without expressing due regards and gratitude to the people involved in this book for their cooperation and patience without which this book would have not been possible.

Rose Nembiakkim

Contents

1

Introduction

Background of the Study

Health is a function, not only of medical care, but also of the overall integrated development of society—cultural, economic, educational, social and political. Each of these aspects has a deep influence on health, which in turn influences all these aspects. Hence, it is not possible to raise the health status and quality of life of people unless such efforts are integrated with the wider effort to bring about the overall transformation of a society (Basu, 1990, 131-142).

Among tribal communities their system of health care has been traditionally prevalent. Though more cultured communities have been exposed to modern medicines, other communities have continued to rely on their traditional systems. They approach human disorders psychosomatically as well as organically, while the modern system aims at bio-chemical efforts.

The traditional health care system are based on a deep observation and understanding of nature and environment. The knowledge of many medicinal plants has been derived through the observation of other animals or other beings in nature.

Different tribal communities also use different plants or different parts of the same plants for particular ailments. This indicates a deep knowledge about these herbs and plants as well as combination and doses of such indigenous objects for cure of different diseases.

The health status of the tribal women is inconceivable in isolation. It is a part of the total tribal health of India. Tribal health by and large is basically eco-dependent. The eco-system and the environment play the most significant role with regard to food, nutrition, immunity and disease process of forest ethnics (Chatterjee, 1993).

Like in any other group, the health aspect of women is very important. In the life of a woman, menarche is a biological phenomenon marking the onset of reproductive age. The reproductive age is also an age when women are the most active.

The status of women in a society is a significant reflection of the level of social justice in the society. Women status is often described in terms of their level of income, employment, education, health and fertility as well as the roles they play within the family, the community and the society. It has been observed that the status of tribal women is comparatively lower than that of tribal men (Ray and Jayanta, 1993).

Health status of tribal women can be ascertained in the light of several parameters, *i.e.*

- Sex ratio,
- Female literacy,
- Marriage practices,
- Age at marriage,
- Fertility, mortality,
- Life expectancy at birth,
- Nutritional status and mother's health,
- Forest ecology,
- Women's health, child bearing and maternal mortality, maternal and child health care practices,
- Family welfare programme, and
- Sexually transmitted diseases and genetic disorders (Basu, 1993, 20).

The level of literacy is undoubtedly one of the most important indicators of social, cultural and health development among the tribal communities.

Literacy is important for the young girl it is correlation with the survival of her children. Infant mortality is found to decrease significantly when the mother is educated up to the primary level or above. The Indian tribes have been exposed to literacy only recently (Mukhopadhyay, 2002, 19).

It is a paradox, however, that the highest female literacy rate (*i.e.* above National average) as well as the lowest is amongst tribal women. One reason for such a paradox is that the tribal women are not a homogenous group although they are known by the generic category 'Tribal women' (Subba and Ghosh, 2003, 296). While the National average of female literacy rate is 29.51 per cent in 1981, the tribal women literacy rate is only 8.04 per cent.

The ground reality is that a majority of them are found in the rural areas were they are disadvantaged in terms of education, occupations etc. Women in the tribal areas are doubly disadvantaged, in the first instance as a tribal and second, as women.

"One of the significant factor regarding tribal female literacy and educational level, is that prior to Independence, a number of tribes came under the influence of Christian missionaries and after embracing Christianity acquired education of sorts" (Mukhopadhyay, 2002, 71).

The focus on women's health has gained impetus in recent times because of new knowledge and a deeper understanding of women's health problems. There is an increasing effort to view women's health issues in a more holistic manner, emphasizing the health needs and concerns of women at every stage and in every aspect of their lives—from birth to old age. A number of programmes and activities have been introduced along with interventions to address women's health issues in the country like the maternity benefits, equal pay for equal work, education in regard to reproductive health etc.

Literature Review

Women in North-East

India has the largest tribal population in the world. It is equal to the sum total of the tribal population of 19 other countries. According to the census, India has a tribal population of 67.8 million, which constitute 8.08 per cent of the total population of India. The tribal groups inhabit different ecological and geo-climatic conditions in different concentrations throughout the country and are distinct biological isolates with characteristic cultural and socio-economic background (Mukhopadhyay, 2002, 1-3).

It is generally believed that tribal women enjoy a high status because their society is egalitarian, they have no *purdah* system, and there is no restriction on women's movement, food habits, and attire and widow re-marriage. Although the status of tribal women is higher as compared to their non-tribal counterparts elsewhere in India, men in their own society do not treat them as equals.

This is one of the most unfortunate aspects of tribal people in the region and factors like education, occupation and religion do not seem to have had any success towards overcoming such gender biases among men. Images of women in the tribal societies are rather negative. Thus, we find proverbs among the Mizos, which states that (a) women's wisdom cannot extend beyond the bank of a river, (b) a wife and an old fence can be replaced anytime and, an unbeaten wife and an uncut weed of the field are both unbearable.

In traditional Garo society, women are ridiculed with the saying that just as a goat is without teeth, so a woman lacks brain. The Mayon Nagas of Manipur considers women as having no principles because they do not have a permanent clan, for their clans' changes into that of their husbands when they marry. Also, among the Zeliangrong Nagas, it is a taboo for a man to sleep with his wife before going to war or going hunting because this may bring bad luck to the whole group (Subba and Ghosh, 2003, 300-302).

Tribal women played a very important role in farming through active participation in shifting cultivation. The arrival of settled farming has marginalized their role. Tribal women also contributed a lot to the family. They are the managers of the house, cooking and providing food for the family members, ensuring drinking water supply and home keeping. A tribal woman occupies an important place in the socio-economic structure of her society. She is found to be exercising a relatively free and firm hand in all aspects related to her social life unlike in the non-tribal societies.

The tribal women in comparison with the women of the caste hierarchy enjoy more freedom in various walks of life. Tribal women belonging to most tribal groups are free to select their life-partners and can also seek and obtain divorce if they are not happy with their husbands. Widow re-marriage is also allowed. Further, the deplorable dowry is not demanded in tribal societies.

A bride-price system prevails under which the bridegroom has to pay money to the parents of the girl whom he wants to marry. The custom of bride-price among the tribes is based on the recognition of the importance of women's role in the economic sphere.

It is the reflection of the fact that women are a productive worker in the economy of the tribe. In case a woman leaves her home after marriage the parents are deprived of a productive worker. Bride price is, therefore, said to be in the form of cash or kind (Mukhopadhyay, 2002, 4-5).

Family planning programmes have been introduced in the tribal areas since the Thrid Five-Year Plan (1961-66).

The status of tribal women in the North-East may also be seen in terms of these four factors:

A. Social Status

(i) Social standing as
—Mother
—Daughter
—Sister
—Wife

(ii) Extent of control enjoyed by women over their lives in social matters
—Marriage
—Divorce
—Family
—Inheritance

B. Economic Condition

(i) Extent of control enjoyed by women in property rights, *e.g.*

—To own property
—To manage property
—To sell property
—To inherit property

(ii) Occupation and livelihood

—To work for a salary and to have control over income
—Distribution of work in the family

C. Political Emancipation

(i) Extent to which women have access to	—Decision Making
(ii) Extent to which women are effectively in position of	—Power

D. Psychological Condition

(i) Attitudes of the society towards women.

(ii) Attitudes of men and women towards women.

(*Source:* Mukhopadhyay, 2002, 5)

The problems of tribal women in the North-East are increasing as tribal life gets disturbed more and more by modern economic development. Due to displacement problems, tribals are giving up their traditional economic pursuits and are migrating to towns and cities to work as labourers. Such tribal labourers, especially women face exploitation and ill-treatment and the change in the economic role is eroding the social status of tribal women.

Lack of educational and training facilities also hampers the progress of tribal women. The rise in literacy rate among women and the improvement in the employment avenues for them are slowly improving the situation. Literacy among the tribal women is 13.62 per cent according to the 1991 census.

If one looks at the condition of tribal women is the North-East at present, it is clear that they have made a lot of progress in almost every field and have been able to enter into many unconventional occupations but if we compare their situation with that of the males in their respective societies, the achievement of women is far from satisfactory.

Whether it is in terms of education, occupation or patriarchal values governing the behaviour of people, women are disadvantaged lot and it may take many years for them before they are able to be at par with men in all respects.

Advent of Missionaries in the North East and the Spread of Education

Durkheim considers education as a social institution that functionally promotes consensus and social integration in new generation through cultivation of those personal quality that can further as a social process (UNESCO, 1969, 228).

Durkheim saw the major function of education as the transmission of society's norms and values. He maintained that, "society can survive only if there exists among its members a sufficient degree of homogeneity; education perpetuates and re-enforces this homogeneity by fixing in the child from the beginning the essential similarities which collective life demands". Without these "essential similarities" cooperation, social solidarity and therefore, social life itself would be impossible.

A vital task for all societies is the welding of a mass of individuals into a united whole, in other words the creation of social solidarity. This involves a commitment to society, a sense of belonging and a feeling that the social unit is more important than the individual (Haralambos with Heald, 1980).

"To become attached to the society the child must feel in it something that is real, alive and powerful, which dominates the person and to which he also owes the best part of himself. Education, and in particular, the teaching of history provides this link between the individual and society. If the history of a society is brought alive to the child, he will want to see he is a part of something larger than himself. He will develop a sense of commitment to the social group (Haralambos with Heald, 1980).

Education is a potent agent not only for the social and psychological changes but it may influence productivity and economic development also, and, that is the reason why for the few years in the literature on development there has been much talk about the relationship between education and economic development and about education as investment (Dubey, 1969).

A look at the tribes of North East India reveals that from the point of view of industrial, technological or agricultural development, all of them are equally backward. But from the literacy point of view, the tribes of this region may be classified into two categories:

(a) "In the first group we may include the Nagas, the Mizo and the Khasis among whom the percentage of literacy is comparatively higher, and, that Christianity has made a marked impact on their way of life.
(b) In the second group—the Mikirs, the Garo, the Bodo, Kachhari, Miri and most of the tribes of the North East Frontier Agency (NEFA) may be included. The percentage of literacy is lower among these tribes and from the view of religion these tribes may be divided into two sub-categories:
    (i) Those professing Hinduism, and
    (ii) Those having faith in the tribal form of worship" (Dubey, 1969).

An analysis of the socio-cultural life of these tribes will show that there is a positive correlation between conversion to Christianity, high percentage of literacy and social change and modernization. The British administration, Christianity and modern education arrived simultaneously in the first quarter of the 19th century in the North East India. The introduction of Christianity resulted certain changes in the structure of the tribal society. Now, the authority of the church assumed higher importance in the religious matters. The missionaries taught the tribals how to read and write. Education brought about a change in their animistic belief. The spread of Christianity is still a continuing process.

The Commissioner of the upper Assam, for the first time, in 1930s wrote to the Government of India to introduce English education in Assam. "English schools were started in Gauhati in the year 1835 and in Sibsagar in the year 1841" (Barpujari, 1965, 275-277). Among the unofficial enterprises, the contribution made by the Christian missionaries to the great vernacular language in Assam, and in the tribal areas in particular, inspired by the zeal of spreading the gospel, was unparalleled.

By 1844 the American Baptist missionaries under Rev. O.T. Culter started as many as 14 schools in the district of Sibsagar (Revenue Procedures in Bengal, 1845).

"The Welsh missionaries who has commenced their activities in the Khasi Jaintia hills also started about half a dozen schools to their credit. Similar institutions were started in Garo hills and Kachhari mohalla in Darang and in 1940 Branson started teaching Bible to the Nagas at Samang along with improved method of manufacturing tea and salt" (Sword, 1840, 61-63).

Spread of Christianity and Education

Before the advent of Christianity, the tribals had a certain concept of religion, they believed in some spirit or powerful being which had its abode in natural objects like stone, river, tree, mountain peak etc. There were many spirits benevolent as well as evil which influenced the life of man.

The spread of Christianity among different sections of the people in the district in the beginning of the 20th century is another achievement in the history of the Churachandpur district. From a small start the district now have a number of Christian organizations as well as missionaries operating in all the corners of the district.

The introduction of Christianity resulted in certain changes in the structure of the tribal society. Now, the authority of the church assumed higher importance in the religious matters. The missionaries taught the tribals how to read and write. Education brought about a change in their animistic belief.

The spread of Christianity is still a continuing process.

- The tribals saw that Christianity would give ghem relief from economic and social oppression.
- They felt that by becoming Christian they would be able to live better lives.
- In the Christian mission they experienced a loving cercern and care which they had not experienced from others.
- They were delivered from their fear of evil spirits.
- They were saved from heavy expenses on sacrifices and feasts.

A number of village surveys conducted by the Census of India (1961) and agro-economic research centre for North East India, Jorhat (Assam) have shown the correlation between

- Christianity and high percentage of literacy, and
- Literacy and social change.

Srinivas concept of 'westernization' may easily be applied to study the nature and extent of change among the tribes of North East India. 'Westernization' refers to the changes brought about in the Indian society and culture as a result of over 150 years of British rule. The term subsuming the changes occurs at different levels of technology, institutions, ideology and values. The influence of westernization among the tribals has been mainly through Christianity.

Christianity spread about in Manipur as a result of the charity work carried out by the British Christian missionaries, which has led to a large-scale conversion of these animistic and supernatural believers, the missionaries facilitated the process of establishing many educational institutions into the region which further led to an increased knwoledge among the tribals.

Cultural Changes and Development

People look at everything in such a positive frame of mind because Christianity provided an ideology that helped the tribal people to maintain their identity in the face of serious erosion of their traditional religious, social and political institutions (Downs, 1983, 185).

Some churches have definitely contributed much towards the preservation of culture. Dances, folk songs, dresses and the like have been integrated for the sacramental of worship and in church functions and at public functions as well. Today, Christian institutions are doing their maximum for the preservation of the cultural identity of the people except in some places where there may be some who are still not aware of the importance of it and may impede its preservation.

To quote the local people, "if Christianity had not arrived in Manipur, it would have been a place full of confusion and contradictions. Only Christianity can save Manipur". Such a statement is made due to the fact that not everything is going on well within the state. Occasional tensions, quarrels and fights occur at different times between different communities. In the last 80 years or so, the missionaries have done a commendable service for the socio-political and economic upliftment of the tribal people.

The development or the changes has occurred because missionary movements are often based on a zeal that is very much philanthrophic. It is true that most of the tribals are still poor, devoid of good education and oppressed by fear which arise out of lack of modern knowledge. But in this respect, they are better off than the poorer class of the non-tribal people due to the fact that the Christian missionaries have worked among the tribals for many years. For many missionaries, their work in their home country is less rewarding than work among the simple and more responsive inhabitants of tribal India (Bose, 1971, 65).

It is an acknowledged fact that a society does not possess that inertia or the potential to change by itself. An external element, a force, an individual or religion has been factors responsible for change of all types.

This is the reason why many scholars rate the impact of missionary endeavours as one of the main agent of cultural, political, social and economic change brought about in Manipur.

In more ways than one the development as well as awareness among the tribals can be attributed to the spread of Christianity among the tribal.

Hence, this brings to light the fact that Christian Missionaries have brought about education in Churachandpur district of Manipur. With the spread of Christianity, education also spread among the Tribals. This brought about a tremendous change in all facets of life among the tribals.

Health Care and the Missionaries

After the missionaries entered the Churachandpur district of Manipur there has been a change in regard to the day to day living routine of the tribal people. Earlier, the foreign missionaries preached the word of God and alongside also mentioned that "Cleanliness is next to Godliness". Many local people joined the missionaries in preaching the word of God and also helped in spreading awareness about the importance of life gifted to mankind by God. Missionaries have introduced the need for maintaining a hygienic lifestyle in order to keep away unwanted illness among the tribal people.

Before the missionaries came to the district the people resorted to sacrifice for curing ill-health and believed in the spirits. However, all these superstitious beliefs have been sidelined after the coming of the missionaries.

Majority of the people had knowledge about the indigenous medicines and even proclaimed to have cured illness. The people who seek care from them were in large number but the number soon declined when the missionaries entered the district with qualified doctors who interacted with the patients. The missionary hospital was one of the first to be established in the Churachandpur district and it was frequented by a large number of people as it was maintained properly. Slowly, few hospitals came up but none could match the missionary hospital and the government hospitals even sometimes use to "borrow" the missionary hospital's operation theatre as they were ill-equipped in comparison to the missionary hospital. The number of people who would consult quacks for any ill-health or rely upon their own and their friends' knowledge regarding care decreased considerably after the provision of health care brought about by the missionaries.

Nevertheless, one can say that the missionaries have been able to bring about a transformation among the tribals of the Churachandpur district. Hygienic style of living have been since then, practiced by the tribals. Care seeking behaviour have also seen an improvement, people now seek care for any ill-health instead of relying upon their own knowledge of care.

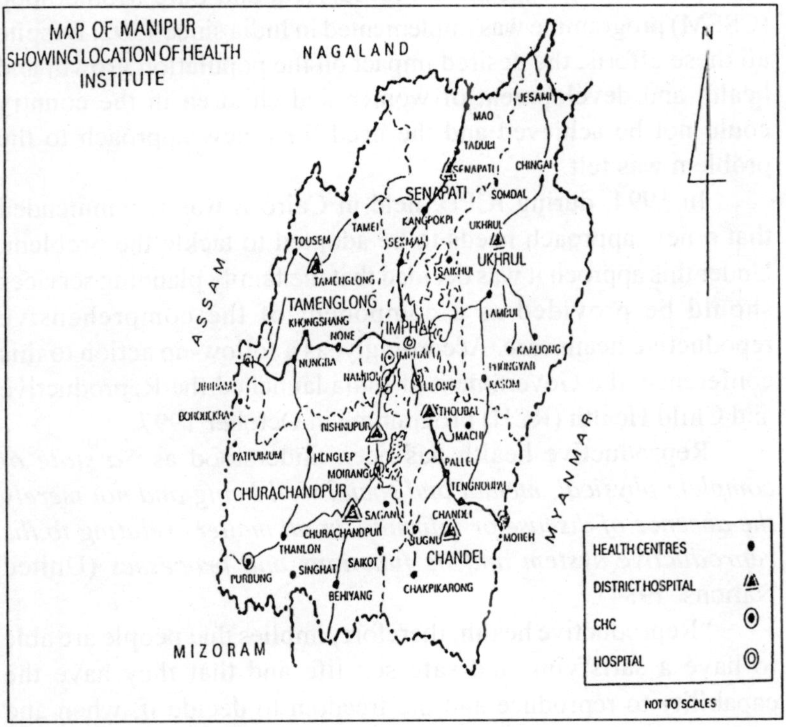

Fig. 1.1: Map of Manipur Showing the Location of Health Institute

Conceptual Framework

Poor health status of women and children in terms of high mortality and morbidity was also another health priority in the country mainly within the North East states. Health facilities like hospitals and health centres were established for providing Maternal and Child Health (MCH) care through ante-natal, pre-natal and post-natal services.

In addition, a number of speical programmes and schemes like immunization against preventable diseases, nutritional interventions, control of diarrhoeal disease etc. were implemented over the past. In order to ensure maximum benefit from these programmes and to provide services in an integrated manner to this vulnerable group, the Child Survival and Safe Motherhood (CSSM) programme was implemented in India since 1992. Despite all these efforts, the desired impact on the population growth and health and development of women and children in the country could not be achieved and the need for a new approach to the problem was felt.

In 1994, during ICPD, held in Cairo it was recommended that a new approach needs to be adopted to tackle the problem. Under this approch it was decided that the family planning services should be provided as a component of the comprehensive repoductive heath care. Accordingly, as a follow-up action to this conference, the Government of India launched the Reproductive and Child Health (RCH) programme in October 1997.

Reproductive health has been understood as *"a state of complete physical, mental and social well-being and not merely the absence of disease or infirmity, in all matters relating to the reproductive system and its functions and processes* (United Nations, 1984).

"Reproductive health, therefore, implies that people are able to have a satisfying and safe sex life and that they have the capability to reproduce and the freedom to decide if, when and how often to do so. Implicit in this last condition are rights of men and women to be informed of and to have access to safe, effective, affordable and acceptable methods of family planning and the right of access to appropriate health care services that will enable the women to go safely through pregnancy and child birth and provide couples with the best chance of having a healthy infant" (ICPD Programme of Action).

The high magnitude of women's reproductive health problems is reflected by the high maternal mortality rate, *i.e.* deaths related to pregnancy and child birth as well as high burden of reproductive morbidity like STI/RTI, gynaecological problems, cancer of the reproductive tract etc.

Safe motherhood programme and the related services components are expected to enable women to go through pregnancy and childbirth safely as well as to ensure survival of the mother (NIHFW, 2000).

The Reproductive and Child Health (RCH) programme is being implemented in India with a major focus on rendering client centred and high quality services to the community. Since women constitute the major client group/users of this programme, greatest attention needs to be given to this group.

The RCH programme was introduced in the state of Manipur in the year 2000. Since its introduction, there has been a certain level of increase in the awareness regarding RCH and its components among the women of Manipur. However, there still remains a portion of women who have not been able to acquire any information about RCH and its facilities. This may be due to the problems of accessibility or its affordability pattern. The majority of the women who are deprived of RCH and its facilities are those belonging to the tribal region in Manipur.

The researcher aims to study the Reproductive Health of the tribal women and how much information they have acquired about the RCH programmes after the arrival of the Christian missionaries as well as the spread of education. More so researcher will study the change pattern in the health seeking behaviour of the tribal and how these changes came about.

Analytical Framework

Two areas selected for study falls within the Churachandpur district of Manipur. They are Lamka town and Takvom village.

Objectives of the Study

1. To draw a profile of the tribal women in the Churachandpur district of Manipur.
2. To examine the socio-cultural factors influencing their reproductive health.
3. To examine the education and health services rendered by the missionaries.

Research Design

The research was undertaken for 45 days.

The study is based on both primary and secondary data. The primary data are the first hand information received from the respondent through interview schedule and observation.

Interview schedule was used to collect information and opinion of the respondent on the basis of a questionnaire prepared earlier. They are mainly the opinion of the women, elders, students with reference to the reproductive health and the role-played by the missionaries. The same set of questionnaire was administered to the women as well as the adolescent group.

Questionnaire was given to the women in Lamka whereas semi-structured interviews, on the basis of the questionnaire, have been held with the women of Takvom. This is because the women of Takvom have not been to school and that they did not know how to read and write English.

In the study area, Lamka town and Takvom village, the researcher has used the grab sampling method to identify the sample population. A total of 30 women from Takvom village and 70 from Lamka town were interviewed. This difference is because the women population in Lamka town is more than the women population in Takvom village. In addition, 65 adolescents were also interviewed (45 girls and 20 boys) in order to know their awareness level about their puberty stage. The adolescent groups were picked conveniently.

In-depth interview with the key informants, *i.e.* the elders to Takvom village and Lamka as well as the District Family Welfare Officer were purposive.

Observation was also used as a tool for collecting data like:

(a) Medical facilities in the area
—Availability
—Accessibility
—Affordability

(b) Transport facility
—Number of vehicles
—Connectivity to the interior village
—Frequency of service

(c) Particular practices, rituals that affect the health seeking behaviour.

Secondary sources were also used, *i.e.* primary census handbook, town and village directory, as well as books written by the local people.

Data Processing

The data collected are processed in simple arithmetical calculation. Tables were prepared with the help of computer for clarity, comparison and interpretation. The tables are interpreted with respect to the overall information and observation received from the respondents, fields and documents.

Chapterisation

This book has been divided into five chapters are as follows:

Chapter 1: Introduction
Chapter 2: Reproductive Health in Family Planning Programme
Chapter 3: The Study Area
Chapter 4: Discussion and Analysis
Chapter 5: Summary and Conclusion

2

Reproductive Health in Family Planning Programme

India's Family Planning Programme

Although India started its official Family Planning Programme way back in 1951, at the time when the programme was initiated in 1952, the concept of small family size norm was non-existent in the country. In fact, India had a unique distinction of being the first country to adopt family planning as an integral part of the socio-economic development plan. For the first time in the history of family planning in India, the Government of India issued on 16th April, 1976 a formal statement entitled "National Population Policy" (Singh, 1976). Clearly, the need at that time was to make people aware about the importance of having a small family, how fertility can be regulated and various aspects of maternal and child health care.

The Janta government issued on 20th April, 1977 a formal policy statement entitled "Family Welfare Programme" (Narain, 1977), replacing the 1976 National Population Policy, they both aimed at achieving the sample objective, namely reduction in the rate of population growth in India.

The 1977 policy statement changed the name of the programme from Family Planning Programme to Family Welfare Programme and that of the ministry from the Ministry of Health and Family Planning to the Ministry of Health and Family Welfare (Reddy, 1994, 86-92).

The 1976 National Population Policy statement and the 1977 Family Welfare Programme statement proposed to pass legislation increasing the age at marriage of girls and boys has multiple benefits. Besides shortening the reproductive span, especially of women, it is likely to develop a sense of responsible parenthood among men and women, and thus create favourable attitudes towards small family norms. Also it improves the health of the mother and child.

The Child Marriage Restraint Act was amended for the third time in 1978 and the minimum age at marriage was increased to 18 for girls and 21 for boys. But marriages of girls below the age of 18 continued, and still continue, to take place.

Family Planning deals with the sensitive area of sexual behaviour and reproduction, which is widely regarded as a personal matter. The strength of a programme, in terms of its implementation, will depend on the amount of inputs available. This refers mainly to the actual availability of institutions (community health centres, primary health centres etc.), personnel (doctors, nurses, health workers etc.) and other physical facilities (building, equipment, medicines, contraceptives etc.).

Greater the magnitude of resources available, better is likely to be the availability of services and the programme. Deployment of resources over different geographic areas can also be important in affecting the process of implementation of the programmes.

Another very important element in the service delivery is the type of follow-up services provided to those who utilize such services. A good follow-up care will enhance the satisfaction of the clients and hence will have a salutary effect on the programme, the type of information, education and communication (IEC) activities undertaken in a programme to popularize the various aspects of child survival and safe motherhood will also be important in creating necessary demand for such services. Thus, the programme gained momentum from the Third Plan onwards with the adoption of Information Education and Communication (IEC) approach.

Link between Family Planning Programme and Reproductive Child Health

"The 1980s saw the emergence of a new perspective on family planning reacting to the earlier emphasis on over-population and projection of women as 'producers of too many babies', members of the international women's health coalition focused on the tendency to neglect other aspects of women's reproductive health. They argued that a reproductive health approach could strengthen existing family planning and health programmes as well as argue dignity and basic rights to women. They identified real location of resources among existing programmes, attention to reproductive health issues of women at all ages, empowerment of women to manage their overall health and sexuality and their participation in policy-making, as central issues. The new paradigm referred to a woman's capability to:

- Understand and enjoy her sexuality by gaining full knowledge of it.
- Regulate her fertility through access to services and information.
- Remain free of reproductive morbidity (and death).
- Bear and raise healthy children." (Qadeer, 2000)

The National Health Policy was introduced in 1983. It emphasized the long-term objective of attaining the replacement level of fertility by the year 2000 (now shifted to 2016). There is a definite concern to strengthen the child survival and safe motherhood programme, the International Conference on Population and Development (ICPD) in Cairo held in 1994 further strengthened the focus on social policies and reproductive health services with a stress on quality (Roy, 1997, 11-22).

The 1994 International Conference on Population and Development held in Cairo has generated widespread commitment to changing family planning programmes from categorical and medically focused service organizations to reproductive health initiatives that embrace a wide range of social and human services.

"The current focus on reproductive health in India marks a global recognition that reproductive health needs have been largely neglected and that the consequences of this neglect have been profound, particularly for women. It also marks the recognition of the need to re-orient India's traditional population programmes to go beyond demographic targets, contraceptive prevalence, and female sterilization, to a more comprehensive focus on reproductive health needs and services, particularly those that respond to Reproductive health needs in ways, which are sensitive to the socio-cultural constraints women, and adolescents, girls face in acquiring services and expressing health needs" (Jejeebhoy, 1999, 16-23).

The currently operating Ninth Five Year Plan seeks to promote reproductive health of women through access to safe and affordable contraceptives, safe management of unwanted pregnancies, services for adolescents, treatment of infertility, initiate male participation and other such related reproductive health services in accordance with the internaitonal conventions. The plan propagates the use of the IEC to ensure responsible reproductive and sexual behaviour, promote awareness about reproductive health needs and optimal utilization of available resources (Government of India, 1997).

The various issues that have to be looked into in order to bring about an improvement in the reproductive health of the women are:

- Safe, effective, affordable and acceptable methods of family planning of choice.
- Safe child bearing and access to appropriate health care services.
- Abortion and access to safe and affordable services.
- The capability to reproduce infertility: we are a culture which prides reproduction, there is little more than anecdotal information on the consequences of infertility for female well-being, preventing her from achieving her desired family size and exposing her to various kinds of emotional distress and harassment or marital disharmony.
- Prevention and care of gynaecological morbidity: other widespread but neglected dimensions of reproductive health in India are gynecological morbidity, notably reproductive tract infections, cervical cell changes and genital prolepses.

- Reproductive health of adolescents, particularly girls: adolescent girls, most of whom are out of school are particularly vulnerable and neglected (Jejeebhoy 1999, 16-23).

"The Government of India had reviewed the National Family Welfare Programme on the basis of various surveys, reports and studies. The important findings are as follows:

1. Targets/incentives distorted the programme implementation: Achievement of targets had become ends in themselves. Disproportionate large portion of the targets (up to 40%) is achieved in the last three months of the financial year instead of the services being provided evenly throughout the years. The targets were set at the State and Central levels (top-down approach) that were never appreciated by the population and health workers at large;
2. Significant gaps existed in infrastructure and in out reach services;
3. Choice of contraceptives was limited;
4. Involvement of males was poor;
5. Involvement of private sector was poor;
6. Quality of services was poor that lead to more complication and generate distrust among users;
7. Low budget allocation resulting in staffing and facility gaps and inadequate package of services;
8. Training and re-orientation programme of staff is not uniform throughout the country. There is hardly any skill development in training; and
9. There is overlapping of Family Planning services."

The Department of Family Welfare after an in-depth sectoral review, undertook many pilot activities to prepare for a total shift in the implementation of the Family Welfare Programme. Such a shift is more likely to address the needs of women who are at risk of unwanted births, and would assist the country to accelerate fertility decline.

India changed the strategy of National Family Welfare Programme to Reproductive and Child Health in 1977 and in the Ninth Five Year Plan (1997-2002) a total change in implementation was recommended" (Kishore, 2002, 17).

Table 2.1: Milestones of Family Welfare Programme

1951-56 (1st Plan)	Family Planning Programme adopted by the Government of India, first of its kind in the world.
1961-66 (3rd Plan)	• Extension Education Approach • Department of Family Planning created in the Ministry of Health • Created Target Oriented Approach • Lippies Loop introduced
1969-74 (4th Plan)	Family Planning services under Primary Health Centre • All India Hospital Post-partum Programme • Medical Termination of Pregnancy (MTP) Act, 1971
1974-79 (5th Plan)	Renaming Family Planning to Family Welfare • Community involvement • Child Marriage Restraint Act, 1978
1983	National Health Policy
1980-85 (6th Plan)	Strengthening of Maternal and Child Health • Strengthening Family Welfare
1985-90 (7th Plan)	Further inclusion of various programmes under MCH
1992-97 (8th Plan)	Child Survival and Safe Motherhood Programme (CSSM)
1993-94	National Development Committee Report • ICPD, Cario, 1994
1996	Target Free Approach Review of the Safe Motherhood Component of CSSM
1997-02 (9th Plan)	Reproductive and Child Health (RCH) (CSSM plus STI and RTI components)

Source: National Health Programme of India, 2002.

Reproductive Child Health Policy and Programmes

Reproductive Health implies that people are able to have a responsible, satisfying and safe sex life and that they have the capability to reproduce and the freedom to decide, if, when, and how often to do so.

This definition focus on right of men and women to be informed of and to have "access to safe, effective, affordable, and acceptable methods of fertility regulation of their choice, and the right of access to appropriate health care services that will enable women to go safely through pregnancy and child birth and provide couples with the best chance of having a healthy infant."

The Essential Components of RCH Programme

They are as follows:

1. Prevention and management of unwanted pregnancy.
2. Maternal care that includes antenatal, delivery and post-partum services.
3. Child survival services for newborns and infants.
4. Management of Reproductive Tract Infaction (RTIs) and Sexually Transmitted Infections (STIs).

Major Elements of RCH Programmes

1. Responsible and healthy sexual behaviour
2. Intervention to promote safe motherhood
3. Prevention of unwanted pregnancies: increase access to contraceptives
4. Safe abortion
5. Pregnancy and delivery services
6. Management of RTI/STD
7. Referral facilities by government/private sector for pregnant woman at risk
8. Reproductive health services for adolescents
9. Screening and treatment of infertility, cancers and other gynaecological disorders (Kishore, 2002, 17-18).

The National Population Policy, 2000 (NPP-2000) affirms the commitment of Government towards voluntary and informed choices and consent of citizens while availing of reproductive health care services, and continuation of the target free approach in administering family planning services.

Table 2.2: Difference in Old and New Approach of Family Welfare Programme

Areas	*Old*	*New*
Primary goal	Meet norms of two child	Still encourage smaller family but help client to meet their own health and family planning goals
Priority Services	Family Planning (sterilization and immunization)	Full range of Reproductive and Child Health services
Performance	Number of cases	Quality of care, satisfaction, coverage measures
Management Approach	Top-down, target driven	Decentralized and client's need based
Attitude to client	Male dominated, motivated, persuade	Gender sensitive listening, assess need, inform, advise
Accountability	To the government system	To the client, community and health and family welfare staff

Source: National Health Programme of India, 2002.

The NPP 2000 provides a policy framework for advancing goals and prioritizing strategies during the next decade, to meet the reproductive and child health needs of the people of India, and to achieve net placement levels (TFR) by 2010. It is based upon the need to simultaneously address issues of child survival, maternal health, and contraception, while increasing outreach and coverage of a comprehensive package of reproductive and child health services by government, industry and the voluntary non-government sector, working in partnership.

3

The Study Area

The health status of the Indian women is extremely low. This is all the more ironic since the primary caregivers of a household's health are women. It may be mentioned that health related studies among the tribal population are found to be limited, most of the available studies being fragmentary in nature without an adequate sample size and standard methodology. There is paucity of studies on many issues affecting the health status of tribal women.

Tribal women in India have specific problems, some of these are built-in problems of these tribal communities and some are imposed upon them, which jeopardize their overall development and progress inclusive of their health. In order to improve the health status of the tribal women, the health care delivery system should be designed for each specific needs and problems by ensuring their personal involvement.

The state of Manipur has about 6.20 per cent of North East India's population in spite of this, the medical facilities are unevenly distributed. There is approximately one doctor per 100 patients. The number of beds in the hospital as well as the dispensaries established is inadequate to meet the health needs of the people. Besides this, big hospital and equipments for specialized treatment as well as specialists are all located in the urban centres.

The health system in the state of Manipur is based upon the primary health care approach as envisaged in the National Health Policy of 1983 with the objective of attainment of "Health for All and All for Health".

The birth rate and death rate of Manipur according to 1999 Statistical Report are given below:

Table 3.1: Birth and death rate of Manipur

	Units	*Rural*	*Urban*	*Total*
Birth rate	Per 1000	19.4	16.4	18.6
Death rate	Per 1000	5.0	6.6	5.4

Profile of Manipur State

The state of Manipur is located in the North-Eastern region of India. It lies between 23.80 degree north and 25.68 degree north latitude to 93.03 degree east and 94.78 degree east longitude.

Manipur state is bounded by the states of Nagaland in the north, Assam in the west and Mizoram and Myanmar in the south-east region. Imphal is the state capital and it lies 790 metres above the sea level.

Table 3.2: Important Statistical Data of Manipur

Total geographical area	22,327 sq. km.
Total population (2001 census)	23,88,634
Male population	12,07,338
Female population	11,81,296
Sex ratio	978
Rural population	18,18,224
Urban population	5,70,410
Density of population (per sq. km)	107
Number of sub-divisions	38
Numbers of community development blocks	34
Number of towns (2001 census)	33

Source: Directorate of Census Operations, Manipur.

Table 3.3: The Composition of the Tribal Group in Manipur

Name of the group	*Population*	*% Share to total population*
Gangte	12793	0.70
Hmar	35767	1.95
Vaiphei	26877	1.46
Paite	40793	2.22
Ralte	250	0.01
Simte	8833	0.48
Thadou	121994	6.64
Zou	168903	0.91

Source: Directorate of Census Operations, Manipur.

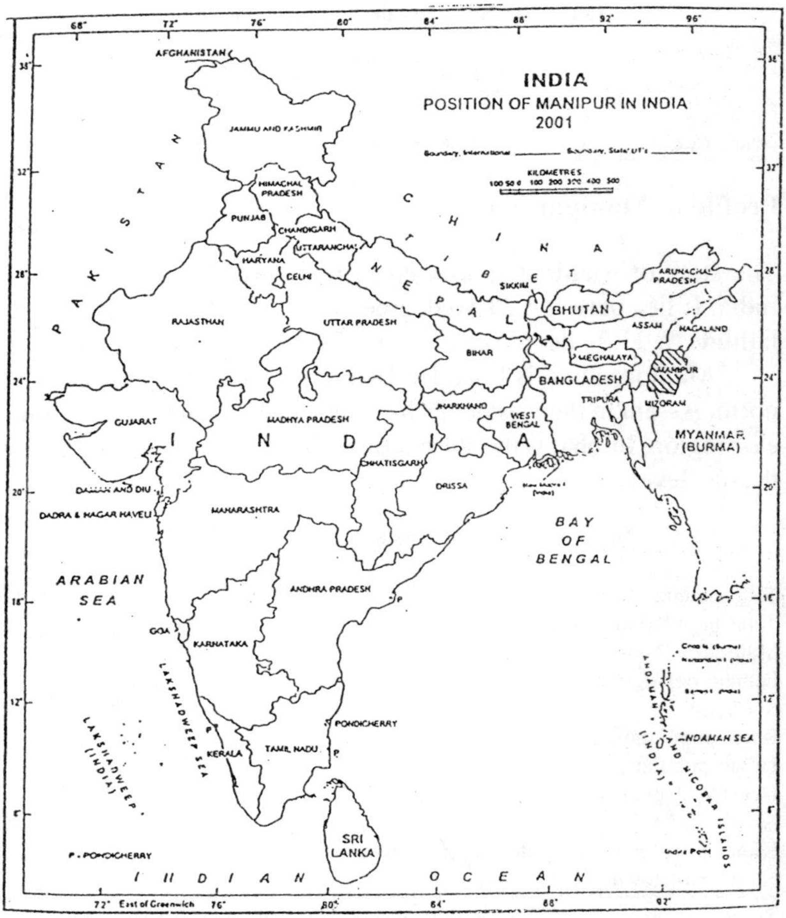

Fig. 3.1: Map of India showing the location of Manipur

In Manipur around 97 per cent of the tribal populations are Christians. The spread of Christianity among different sections of the people in the district in the beginning of the 20th century is another achievement in the history of the Churachandpur district. From a small start the district now have a number of Christian organization as well as missionaries operating in all the corners of the district.

Table 3.4: Religionwise Distribution of Population

Christianity	1,64,453
Hinduism	9,925
Islam	1,248
Sikhism	192
Jainism	14
Buddhism	04
Other religion and persuasion	347
Religion not stated	01

Source: Directorate of Census Operations, Manipur.

The introduction of Christianity resulted in certain changes in the structure of the tribal society. Now, the authority of the church assumed higher importance in the religious matters. The missionaries taught the tribals how to read and write. Education brought about a change in their animistic belief. The spread of Christianity is still a continuing process.

The study covers Churachandpur. It has been purposefully chosen for the following reasons:

1. It is a hill district where the missionaries have played an active role in bringing about awareness regarding the importance of education.
2. No empirical study has been done in the area of the awareness regarding reproductive health by the Paite women.

About Churachandpur

The district (Churachandpur) was created as Manipur south district on 12th November 1969 and it was re-christened as Churachandpur district, named after Churachand Singh the then Maharaja of Manipur on the 15th July 1983.

The total geographical area of Churachandpur district is 4570 sq.km with a population of 2,28,707 according to the 2001 census. The whole of the district area is hilly and the average altitude of the district is 914 metres above the mean sea level and the height of the hill ranges spread from a minimum of 200 metres to a maximum of 2109 metres.

Table 3.5: Climate

Maximum temperature	39 degree Celsius
Minimum temperature	0 degree Celsius
Maximum humidity	100%
Minimum humidity	58%

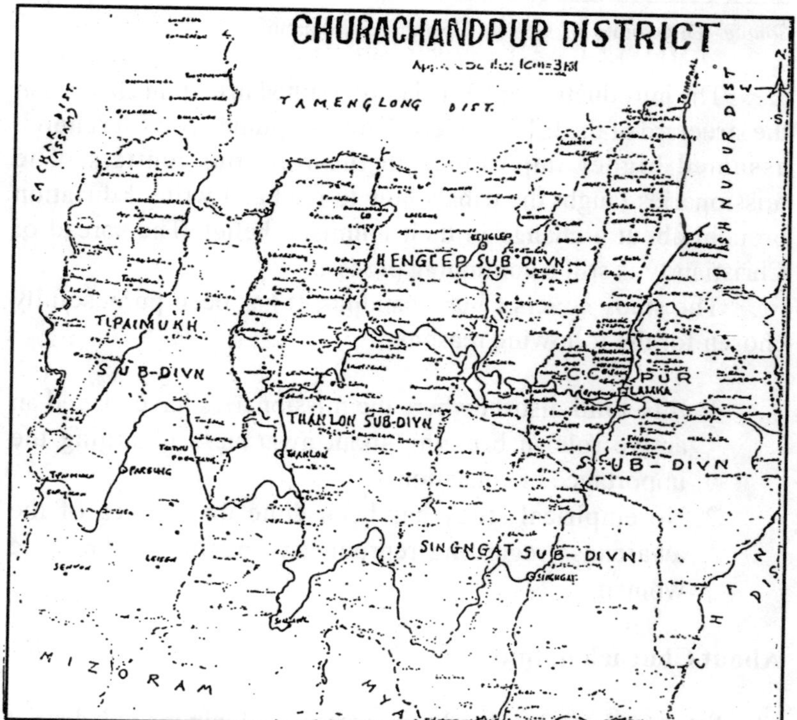

Fig. 3.2: Map of Manipur showing the Location of the Study Area: Churachandpur District

Churachandpur district is divided into five-administrative/ revenue sub-divisions, they are:

Tipaimukh sub-division
Thanlon sub-division

Henglep sub-division
Singngat sub-division
Churachandpur sub-division

The district headquarter, *i.e.* Churachandpur is better known as 'Lamka' for the local people, it is 65 kms away from the state capital—Imphal and is well connected by road and it takes hardly two hours to cover the distance.

Population

Churachandpur district is mostly inhabited by the Chin-Kuki-Mizo-Zomi ethnic group of people which comprises around 14 tribes like the Hmar, Paite, Simte, Thadou, Zou, Lushai, Ralte, Sukte, Gangte, Kom, Aimol, Chiru, Chothe, Vaiphei etc. and the other tribes and communities like the Kabui, 'Pangal' (Muslim), Meitei, Bengalis, Biharis etc. "But there are no communication problems as people understand each of the dialects spoken and that is why Churachandpur is called the 'Pentecostal town'—it is often compared to Jerusalem in A.D. 33 when the Holy Spirit came upon the apostles and the language they spoke was understood by people speaking as many as 15 different dialects" (Hatzaw, 2003, 61).

The total population of Churachandpur district as per 2001 census (provisional) was 2,28,707 out of which 1,14,740 are males and 1,13,967 were females. The sex ratio was 993 and with a population density of 50 per sq.km. The sub-division or distributions of population according to their tribes, castes, other communities, religion, sex rato and decadal growth percentage rate of population are given below:

Table 3.6: Scheduled Tribe Population of Churachandpur District

Total Population	1,64,709
Male	83,760
Female	80,949
Percentage to Total Population of District	93.49%

Table 3.7: Scheduled Caste Population of Churachandpur District

Total Population	301
Male	210
Female	91
Percentage to Total Population of District	0.17%

Table 3.8: Other Population

Total Population	11,174
Male	6,987
Female	4,185
Percentage to Total Population of District	6.34%

Table 3.9: Sex Ratio in Churachandpur District

Year	*Sex Ratio*
1951	1048
1961	1004
1971	976
1981	929
1991	931
2001	993

Table 3.10: Decadal Percentage Growth Rate of Population

Year	*Population Percentage Decadal*
1951-1961	46.20
1961-1971	57.19
1971-1981	37.37
1981-1991	30.72
1991-2001	29.85

Source: Directorate of Census Operations, Manipur.

Literacy and Education

The literacy rate of the Manipur state as a whole is 68.87 per cent (male—77.87% and female—59.70%) according to 2001 census.

Total literacy rates have improved over time in Churachandpur district.

The following tables show the total literate population and the changes in the literacy rate in the district according to 2001 census.

Table 3.11: Total Literate Population Percentage in Churachandpur District

(in per cent)

Male	84.98
Female	64.40
Total	**74.67%**

Source: 2001 Census.

Table 3.12: Change in Literacy Rate in Churachandpur District

(in per cent)

Year	*Male*	*Female*	*Total*
1991	66.38	49.30	58.17
2001	84.98	64.40	74.67

Source: 2001 Census.

Educational Institutions

There has been an increase in the number of private educational institutions in the district during the last five to ten years. They are mostly English medium schools and colleges offering courses up to higher secondary level. The government and government-aided schools are the primary and the basic education providers to the rural villages.

Table 3.13: Educational Institutions in the District

Primary Schools	293
Junior High Schools	1214
High Schools	69
Higher Secondary Schools	07
College	02

Source: Zonal Education Officer, Churachandpur.

The tribes of the North-East India feel greatly indebted to the missionaries from the West for their work of uplifting them.

There is, therefore, a feeling of close relationship, if not loyalty, to the people who brought them the benefits of education and social and economic advancements.

The researcher has taken Takvom village (rural) and Lamka (urban) which are within the Churachandpur district, in order to collect the primary data.

Takvom Village

Takvom is a village, which is inhabited mainly by the Paite tribe. There are approximately 70 households in the village and a population of about 700. The village is approximately 25 kms far from the district Lamka. The roads connecting Takvom to the other areas is rough. During rainy season it is very muddy and dusty during the dry season. It is a *kuccha* road. There is no transportation available. The village people commute from one place to the other by walking. Private vehicle also finds it difficult to enter the village, as the roads are very narrow.

Majority of the inhabitants of the village are engaged in agriculture.

Between 1996 and 1998 there was in ethnic clash between the Kuki and the Paite in the whole district of Churachandpur. Takvom was also affected and due to this, houses of the Paite tribe were burnt and many were forced to leave the village as a result of which there are at present about only 45 households with a population of approximately 365 people. Many people have also migrated to other villages in search of better living condition. However, there were 4 houses being constructed again during the researcher's study. The entire population of Takvom follows Christianity as a religion and belongs to the Evangelical Baptist Convention (EBC). There is only one Church in the entire village.

In Takvom village the houses are built from bamboo and wood. There are no *pucca* houses in the village. There is no electric supply in the village (See Fig. 3.3).

There is sacarcity of water because there is no well water and the villagers depend upon spring water for drinking and other purposes. For this, they have to walk at least 3 to 4 kms to fetch water.

Each household have small landholdings in which ginger and rice is cultivated and is used for their own consumption or sold in the nearby villages. Pig and cow is the main livestock reared by the villagers. During festive season and other occasions cows and pigs are in high demand and it gets them a good price.

Takvom village does not have any health/medical facilities in the village. For major health problems they go to the district hospital, Lamka. However, there are still few people in Takvom who resort to the indigenous method of health care.

Majority of the people of Takvom village are unemployed, many take to farming and rearing domestic animals or going to the town in search of daily wages.

The literacy rate in the village is very low, only a few of them know how to read the Bible as well as write letters but only in the local dialect, that is Paite. There is only one junior high school up to class 8, which is under the zonal education officer ironically, there is no school building.

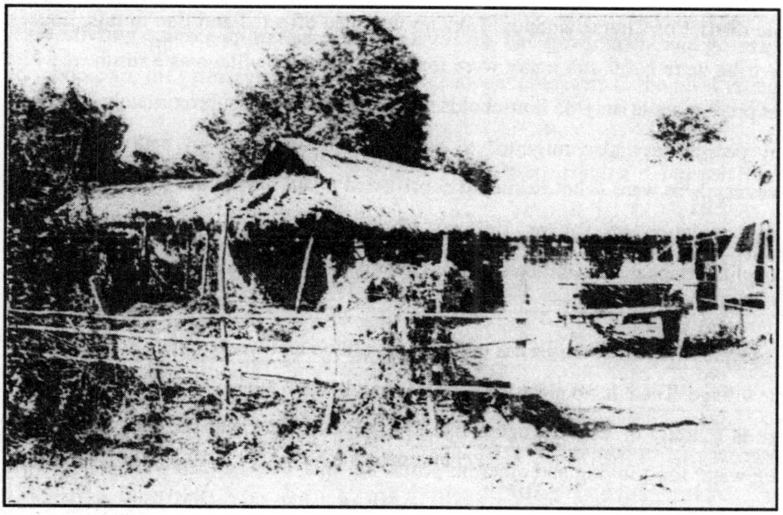

A View of a house in Takvom Village made of Bamboo and Straw

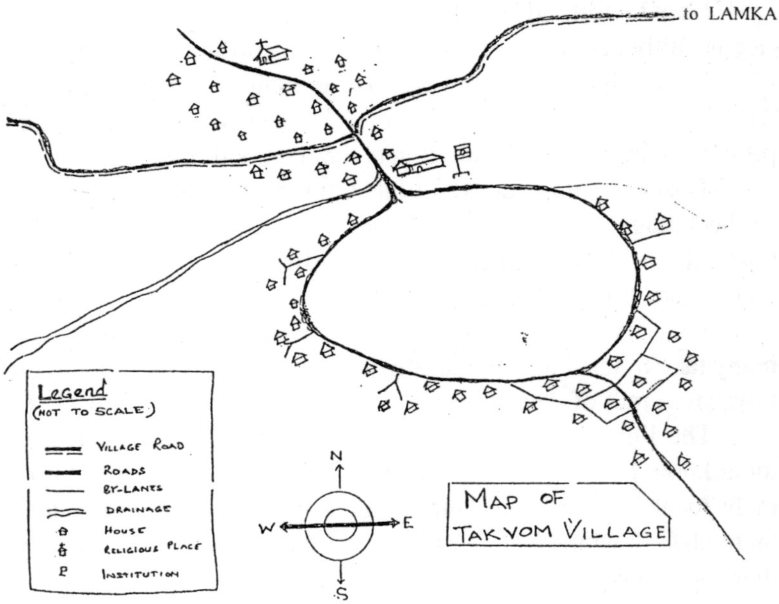

Fig. 3.3: Map of Takvom Village (National Map)

Lamka Town

Lamka is 65 kilometres away from the state capital, Imphal. It has a population of nearly 2,28,707 (2001 census). Majority of the population in Lamka belongs to the Paite tribe although other tribes such as Hmar, Zou, Lushai, Simte, Vaiphei, Meitei also reside in Lamka besides the ımagrants mainly from Bihar and Bengal.

Compared to Takvom Village it is very much developed. For the villagers Lamka is a town of "opportunities". There is no problem of transport facility within Lamka because all the local buses and state buses leave from the town.

There are 2 colleges in Lamka and 129 primary schools, 43 junior high schools and 38 senior high schools. Majority of the schools are private schools having affiliation with one or the other church or supported by foreigners abroad. According to the 2001 census, the literacy rate is 74.67 per cent.

Many families have tap water supply in their house whereas others have to fill water from the well or the pipe water that flow only for one to two hours.

The district hospital and other important state government offices are located within Lamka. Majority of the Lamka population are employed in the State and Centre Government offices and there are many officers in the town from IAS, IPS, SDO, to doctors, lecturers, teachers as well as businessmen and petty shop owners.

There are also many Non-Governmental Organizations working in Lamka. The focus area of the NGOs is rehabilitation of the drug users. Many of the NGOs receive their funds from the foreign agency that are mostly associated with the church.

The majority of the population in Lamka are Christian by religion, however, the Christians are divided into different churches on the basis of their Christian faith. There are about 35 different churches in Lamka.

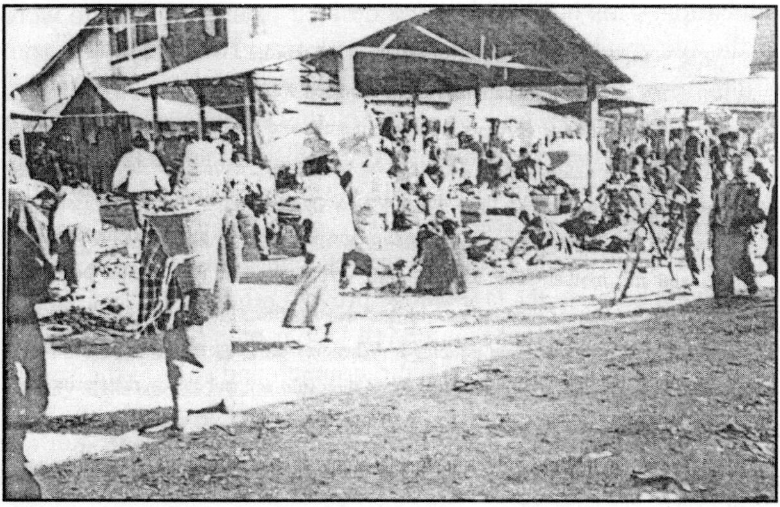

Lamka Town

This picture is the Market Place of Lamka Town. Home grown vegetables are sold here early in the morning by the women from other villages.

4

Discussion and Analysis

Since the researcher is involved in the study of RCH, her respondent are females. The average age taken in both Lamka and Takvom are between 25 to 50 yrs. Adolescent (both male and female) belonging to the age group of 16 to 18 yrs have been taken for the study.

The following is the finding of the researcher about the reproductive health status of the women before the spread of education. This information was derived from women who were in the age group of 55 to 65 years, both from Lamka and Takvom village.

In relation to reproductive health the women were very much ignorant about their own health aspect and also lacked information about pregnancy, delivery as well as the care of the infants and the mother. The women were very shy when they would become pregnant. They would cover themselves with shawls and other cloth to hide the bulge in the stomach to prevent others from noticing it. Whenever the pregnant women felt labour pain the village priest (*siampu*) would blow air on their stomach and call on the spirits for healing. How effective it is, is not yet known.

Birth of the child during those days would take place anytime and anywhere. Many of the women have had delivery while working in their fields or while fetching water. When childbirth takes place the baby is cleaned only with water after which no cleaning takes place for a long time. The umbilical cord of the baby would be tied with a thread and cut apart by a sharp small bamboo strip and kept inside a small basket weaved for the cord only. It is not thrown but kept inside the basket till the blood drips dry and becomes rotten. However, there is no significance attached to the mentioned practice.

The feeding process of the child was not at all hygienic. The mother would first eat "zuha" (rice beer) to soften them and then feeds the infant.

Moreover the women were not aware about any other kind of reproductive ill health problems. The only problems they were aware were like the vaginal discharge, irritation as well as unable to urinate properly. They, at the same time never took medical help for it as they thought that since it happens to everyone it is normal.

Table 4.1: Age Composition of Women Respondents of Takvom Village and Lamka Town

Age	*Takvom Village*	*Lamka*	*Total*
25-35	18	27	45
35-45	9	30	39
45+	3	13	16
Total	**30**	**70**	**100**

Source: Field Survey, 2003.

In keeping with the sample population of 100 women, 30 women from Takvom and the remaining 70 women from Lamka were interviewed. More women from Lamka were interviewed because Lamka have more population than Takvom village.

The females in the Takvom village were easily available for interview because they were not employed and worked in the fields nearby or were doing household chores. However, majority of the women in Lamka were employed in the State and Centre Government offices as teachers, lecturers, doctors etc. Few of them were housewives.

Table 4.2: Age Composition of the Adolescent Group

Age	*Boys*	*Girls*	*Total*
16-18	20	45	65

Source: Field Survey, 2003.

The researcher has combined the data of the adolescent group in both the Takvom village and Lamka as the student respondent of Takvom goes to schools in Lamka and their information about puberty and health are in the same line as the students of Lamka. Here, the researcher interviewed students who had taken up different discipline in order to compare whether there was any influence of their subject in their knowledge about health and puberty.

The Takvom Village Women

Takvom is a remote village, which is inhabited mainly by the Paite tribe. The village is approximately 25 kms far from the district, Lamka. Takvom has approximately 70 households and a population of about 700. The roads connecting Takvom to the other areas is rough. During rainy season it is very muddy and dusty during the dry season. It is a *kuccha* road. There is no transportation available.

The village people commute from one place to the other by walking. Private vehicle also finds it difficult to enter the village, as the roads are very narrow. For minor illness they do not go out of the village but regarding major illness they go to the district hospital as it is the nearest hospital to their village and it is affordable for them as the district hospital is a government run hospital.

When asked about the physical changes regarding the adolescent stage the women were able to inform the researcher about the physical changes, which both males and females undergo once they reach puberty, they mentioned the following criteria for females:

- Enlargement of breast,
- Menstrual cycle begins,
- Pimples come out,
- Face structure undergoes a slight change etc.

For males the following criteria were given:

- Voice begins to crack,

- Moustache develops,
- Pimples come out etc.
- Enlargement of the genital

Although they have not received any formal information on this their knowledge is entirely dependent on their experience. The women further mentioned that they were not informed about the menstrual cycle by anyone, they became aware about it when it occurred to them. Only few of them mentioned that they had knowledge about it from their peer group. They informed the researcher that prior knowledge is important, as they were frightened when it occurred to them, they felt as if something was wrong with them and that they were about to die. All the women in the village use cloth for menstrual flow. Earlier they would just drape two to three "puanteng" (*traditional cloth wrapped around the waist*) in order to hide the stain. After washing it and then drying it in the sun, many of them re-use the menstrual cloth. They further mentioned that they are not ashamed to dry it in the open because all the women dry it in the open and it is a known fact that every woman has a menstrual cycle.

However, the women who have now become mothers and are of a younger generation informed the researcher that they would be telling their daughters about menstrual cycle once they attained puberty. When asked about the ready made pads available in the market they all did not want to use it as it was too expensive for them and moreover they have got used to using the cloth.

Religion further does not pose a problem for them and during their menstrual cycle they attend the Sunday service. They do not feel ashamed to go to church as having menses is not a sin and they also continue doing their chores, as it does not hinder them from their routine work.

The women in the village were also not aware of the reproductive organs. However, majority of them knew about reproductive ill-health problems such as vaginal discharge, irritation etc. because they have experienced it. Since in the village many women suffer from the same problem they did not regard it as a health hazard and do not take medical care for it instead they would take care themselves by washing their vagina with "tangal", (*local name for a syrup made from ash and soda, which is edible*).

On questions regarding delivery, the elderly women informed the worker that there were times when they use to have children in the fields without any support. They would continue to work during pregnancy and when the time comes delivery would just take place. However, among the women who are between the age group of 25-35, few of them had delivery in the district hospital and the remaining had delivery from the local *dais.*

Regarding the Family Life Education, the respondents felt that school is an institution that teaches everything and they held school teachers in high esteem. However many were against the introduction of sex education in the school as they felt that the student will be encouraged to go the 'wrong way'. They even said that the children should be send to school as they learn a lot of things not only from the school but even from their peer groups since they spend maximum time with their friends.

Ironically, very few of the respondent's children go to school in Lamka. Their children do not stay in the village but are staying with their relatives in Lamka, as commuting from Lamka to Takvom everyday was not possible. Many of them wanted to send their children to school but they could not afford the education of their children.

The tables inform us about the *Takvom Village Women* and their access to information and knowledge regarding the different aspects of health and health care and whether there has been an involvement of the missionaries in this regard.

In the following tables the *Missionary sources* include: the local pastor, Church youth group, Church women's group, Church literature.

The *non-missionary sources* include: the government health workers, doctors and nurses, NGOs working in the specific field, volunteers of different NGOs and peer groups.

In Takvom village there is no missionary hospital, however, there are visiting doctors and health workers from both the government and the missionary Hospitals as well. In Lamka town there is 3 missionary hospitals and 4 government hospitals.

The table below reflects that the village women in majority sought care for their ill-health from the non-missionary hospital. This includes mainly the private run clinics in the town (Table 4.3). The major ill-health experienced by the village women of Takvom is the viral fever. Surprisingly none of the women in the village seek care from the missionary run hospital whenever they experienced typhoid (Table 4.3).

Table 4.3: Health Seeking Services

Type of Ill-health Experienced	*Care Sought from*		*Total*
	Missionary hospital	*Non-missionary hospital*	
Malaria	1	3	
Diarrhea	2	4	
Viral Fever	4	9	
Typhoid	0	4	
Jaundice	1	2	
Total	**8**	**22**	**30**

Source: Field Survey, 2003.

The women of Takvom village preferred the services of a non-missionary hospital as against the missionary hospital (Table 4.4). Majority of them would also like to go outside Manipur for seeking care services if given an opportunity but as of now not many can think about going beyond the capital, Imphal. According to them, most of the non-missionary hospitals are private and cater to the people efficiently and this information has been passed on to them from their friends who had sought care from the non-missionary hospitals.

Table 4.4: Care Services Utilization

Utilized Care Services	*Preferred Services of*		*Total*
	Missionary hospital	*Non-missionary hospital*	
Inside Manipur	5	6	
Outside Manipur	4	15	
Total	**9**	**21**	**30**

Source: Field Survey, 2003.

The Takvom village women have acquired information pertaining to menstrual cycle from the missionaries though the number of the women who gained information from them is less in comparison to those who derived the information from the non-missionary source (Table 4.5). Information regarding RTI/STI and its prevention and causes was mainly derived from the non-missionary sources like the hospital nurses, friends circle as well as through the various advertisements taken out by the health department of Manipur (Table 4.5).

Table 4.5: Knowledge about Reproductive Health

Information Pertaining to:	*Source of Information from the*		*Total*
	Missionaries	*Non-missionaries*	
Menstrual Cycle	5	15	
RTI/STI: Its causes and prevention	1	9	
Total	**6**	**23**	**30**

Source: Field Survey, 2003.

The Takvom village opined that the missionaries did not contribute their knowledge in regard to the reproductive health programmes. Majority of them mentioned that they acquired information regarding immunization during pregnancy only from the non-missionary sources, district hospital nurses and expectant mothers (Table 4.6). They also mentioned that they have received information about the small family norm from the various hoardings put up by the health department in and around the district.

Table 4.6: Knowledge of Reproductive Health Programmes

Knowledge Experienced	*Source of information from*		*Total*
	Missionaries	*Non-missionaries*	
Small Family Norm	0	6	
Anti-Natal Care	0	2	
Immunization during Pregnancy	0	17	
Identification of high risk pregnancy	0	5	
Total	**0**	**30**	**30**

Source: Field Survey, 2003.

Very few of them acquired information regarding the ante-natal care and not much information was received regarding the identification of high risk pregnancy even from the non-missionary hospital (Table 4.6).

In this table one can see that the missionaries did not contribute to the supply of the contraceptives among the women of the Takvom village. Majority of the women use the condom method of contraceptive (Table 4.7). This could be mainly because of the easy availability as well as usage of the condom. The next common contraceptive used among the Takvom women is the oral pills.

Very vew of the women have gone in for total sterilization and none of the women interviewed in the village have ever had abortion (Table 4.7). They informed the researcher that abortion was against their religious belief as it involved killing an urborn child.

Table 4.7: Utilization of Contraceptives

Type of Contraceptives Used	*Source of Supply from*		*Total*
	Missionary hospital	*Non-missionary hospital*	
Vasectomy	0	3	
Tubectomy	0	4	
Total Sterilization	0	2	
IUCD	0	4	
Oral Pills	0	7	
Condoms	0	10	
MTP	0	0	
Total	**0**	**30**	**30**

Source: Field Survey, 2003.

The missionaries have enabled the Takvom women to understand the importance of hygiene. This information has percolated down to them from their parents who were informed by the missionaries. They mentioned that the missionaries laid emphasis on keeping the house clean (Table 4.8). According to them they have also made provision of a toilet as compared to earlier times when they would go and do it in the open fields. The

Takvom village women have been informed about the storage of drinking water from both the missionary and the non-missionary sources (Table 4.8).

Table 4.8: Awareness Regarding Hygiene

Awareness Regarding	*Source of Information from the*		*Total*
	Missionaries	*Non-missionaries*	
House Cleanliness	10	5	
Toilet Facility	5	4	
Storage of Drinking Water	3	3	
Total	**18**	**12**	**30**

Source: Field Survey, 2003.

From the table below we can see the the Missionaries did spread some information regarding nutrition (Table 4.9). But more inputs were received from the non-missionaries (Table 4.9). Regarding the consumption of meat in the village, many of them informed the researcher that the staple diet includes meat even it was a small piece. Especially in the winters meat is preferred. Regarding the caloric intake of food as well as follow of a food routine the women of Takvom village felt that they got their information from the health workers who would visit the village once in a while (Table 4.9).

Table 4.9: Awareness Regarding Nutrition

Awareness in Terms of	*Source of Information from*		*Total*
	Missionaries	*Non-missionaries*	
Caloric intake of an individual	3	4	
Non-vegetarian diet	6	10	
Follow of Food Routine	1	6	
Total	**10**	**20**	**30**

Source: Field Survey, 2003.

The above table reflects that, of the total women interviewed in Takvom village, majoirty of them felt that the Missionaries did not do much in changing their health status (Table 4.3). The women in the village said that they preferred to access the health services provided by the district hospitals as well as the private clinics (Table 4.4) and the knowledge regarding seeking care during ill-health have been brought forward by the early missionaries who give this information to their mothers.

There was no Missionary intervention regarding Reproductive Health Programmes. There was not a single woman who mentioned the Missionaries role in the awareness about Reproductive Health Programmes (Table 4.6). Awareness regarding RH programmes was spread by the government through the means of posters, billboards, pamphlets as well as through advertising in the local channels. Nevertheless, majority of the women felt that the missionaries have brought about a change in their living practices by spreading information pertaining to hygiene and also nutrition (Table 4.8 and Table 4.9).

The missionaries have also been instrumental in not only bringing about educational facilities in this small village but also in developing an interest for learning among the people. Majority of the woman do not deny that it was the missionaries only who brought in education and thereby setting up schools in the village (Table 4.10). The women also expressed that many private schools are located within the town because of profit motives and hence one finds only missionary/Government school in the village.

Table 4.10: Criteria for a School

Criteria for School	*School Preferred*		*Total*
	Missionary	*Non-missionary*	
English Medium	7	5	
Qualified Teachers	8	2	
Quality of Teaching	6	2	
Total	**21**	**9**	**30**

Source: Field Survey, 2003.

Many of the women were of the opinion that the quality of education/teaching in the missionary school is far better than any government schools (Table 4.10), also most of the non-missionary schools resort to the local dialect during teaching and hence there is not much scope for the student to learn English whereas it is not so in the missionary schools (Table 4.10). This may be because missionary school teachers are more serious about their work whereas the government employees just enter the school to collect their monthly salary.

Women of Lamka Town

The population of the Lamka town is approximately 2,28,707. There are a number of people who are employed in the state as well as Centre Government offices, this reflects that the literacy rate among the people of Lamka is high (Table 3.11 and Table 3.12).

Moreover, there are a number of women who are working in different positions under the State or Central Government. There are also businesswomen as well as petty shop owners. Many of the women who are working have gone to school till the standard of class eight. The respondents were aware of the physical changes which both the male and the female undergo as they reach puberty. Among the respondents there were only 5 out of the 70 women who could define puberty by virtue of them being a doctor, nurse as well as teachers.

All of them were of the opinion that as puberty sets in there is a change of voice for the males and their moustache starts to grow whereas for the females, one can see that there is an enlargement of their breast as well as their menstrual cycle begins. Pimples are a common sight in both the males and the females during puberty. The information that is derived from Lamka women is not slightly different from that information acquired from Takvom village. This may be due to the fact that the urban women also have had no formal education and that their information is based mainly on experiences and observations.

Out of the 70 women interviewed only few of them did not have prior knowledge about the menstrual cycle whereas most of them were informed about the menstrual cycle either by their mothers or through sharing it among their friends circle. All the women interviewed were aware of the duration of their menstrual cycle and if irrigularity occurs then they blamed it on their ill health.

Many of the women started using the pads (sanitary napkins) during their menstrual cycle recently. They were aware about these pads from the television commercials. Those who have changed their preference from cloth to the readymade pads find it very useful and not troublesome. The most famous pads in Lamka during the researcher's visit was *"SHE"* which was imported from Moreh, Burma. For disposing of the pads they burn it or wrap it in a paper and throw it. Till now some of the women continue to use clothes during the menstrual cycle. As they have become accustomed to it and feels that pads are for the younger females.

After the cloth is utilized they wash it and re-use it for the next cycle. They have no qualms in drying the menstrual cloth in the sun just like the women of Takvom. The cloth is changed after every two months.

They also attend the church service during the cycle and do not feel ashamed. If they ever happen to miss the church service during the menstrual cycle then it would not be because of them feeling dirty but only because of the cramps and stomach ache which some of the women undergo during those stage.

To the question regarding reproductive health, the women who were more educated were aware of the reproductive organs whereas majority of them did not know anything about the reproductive organs but simply mentioned that it is an organ for the various processes of reproduction.

Majority of the women were aware of the reproductive ill-health problems such as the vaginal discharge, irritation, itching pain, irregular menses etc. Some of the women have not experienced any of the ill-health problems and the women who experienced irritation as well as vaginal discharge seek care from the district hospital.

However none of the respondents informed the researcher about the reproductive tract infections. The researcher feels that there are two possibilities:

1. They do not know what is the reproductive tract infection.
2. They do not feel comfortable to divulge such information to anyone.

All of the women interviewed have heard about the reproductive health programmes. The medium of their information is:

- Casual conversation with friends/neighbours
- Media: newspaper, television, radio
- Awareness campaign around the area
- Hospital billboards
- Through the doctors themselves.

Majority of the women in Lamka town have had used contraceptives at a certain period of time. These contraceptives are available in all the chemist stores in and around Lamka. Most of the women interviewed have used the temporary method of birth control that includes oral pills, condoms and only few of the women have gone in for permanent sterilization. The reason for adopting the permanent birth control is as follows:

- Due to the health problem of the woman
- Cannot maintain a large family (small family is a happy family)
- Want to give the best to the children

When asked about the importance of family life education, many of the women felt that now, when the children are exposed to a more different lifestyle through the medium of television and the variety of programmes it airs. It is indeed important for the school to make the students aware about the various facets of life as their parents cannot always monitor them.

They feel that students who are especially in the higher classes of 11 and 12 should be exposed to sex education on the large scale as the case of unwanted pregnancy is also on the rise in Lamka and casual relationship among the students will not be promoted.

Moreover with the deadly disease AIDS/HIV student should be made more aware.

Apart from sex education they also feel that information regarding family values, importance of being educated should be given. The women also informed the researcher that as a parent they never held discussion regarding sexuality and reproduction with their adolescent children. They feel that it is necessary but at the same time feel embarrassed to take up the issue with their adolescent children. They also opined that informant about reproduction and sexuality is shared among the friends circle.

When the women group was asked whether the spread of education have played a part in bringing about change in regard to the health aspect, they all felt that education have brought about more awareness among the tribal people. They said that though the missionaries laid the foundation for education by setting up educational institutions that further continued the process of disseminating information and bring about awareness among the people. The presence of the missionaries in the town itself was a motivating factor for the people because they started to follow the lifestyles of the foreign missionaries.

Regarding the health status, they attributed the role played by the missionaries because the health of the people has seen a tremendous change. Earlier, for any kind of health care they would resort to the practices done by the "siampu" but now, due to the spread of awareness about the various kinds of ill health and their care they prefer to go to the doctors.

Immunization was also not prevalent until recently before it was introduced the women were not aware that the infants have to be immunized even before birth. Jokingly they commented that without being immunized they are still alive and without major ill health problems and in contrast the children who are being immunized are suffering from a lot of ill health problems.

In the following tables the *Missionary sources* includes: the local pastor, Church youth group, Church women's group, Church literature.

The *non-missionary sources* includes: the government health workers, doctors and nurses, NGOs working in the specific field, volunteers of different NGOs and peer groups.

In Takvom village, there is no missionary hospital, however, there are visiting doctors and health workers from both the government and the missionary Hospitals as well. In Lamka town there is 3 missionary hospitals and 4 government hospitals.

The tables inform us about the *Lamka town women* and their access to information and knowledge regarding the different aspect of health and health care and whether there has been an involvement of the missionaries in this regard.

The Lamka town women generally sought care for their ill-health in the non-missionary hospital (Table 4.11). Majority of the women have had experienced viral fever just like the women of the Takvom Village (Table 4.3). For the various ill-health experienced by the women (Table 4.11), most of them informed the researcher that they sought care for the illness in the non-missionary hospitals. Diarrhea was another ill-health problem commonly experienced by the Lamka town women.

Table 4.11: Health Seeking Services

Type of Ill-health Experienced	*Care Sought from*		*Total*
	Missionary hospital	*Non-missionary hospital*	
Malaria	2	8	
Diarrhea	5	12	
Viral Fever	8	21	
Typhoid	1	5	
Jaundice	3	5	
Total	**19**	**51**	**70**

Source: Field Survey, 2003.

During illness a majority of the Lamka women preferred to go to the non-missionary hospital. Also, the number of women who seek care from the non-missionary hospital which is outside the state of Manipur is more as compared to the women who would seek care from the non-missionary hospital inside Manipur (Table 4.12). Within Manipur many good hospital both private and Government have opened up in the recent years.

Table 4.12: Care Services Utilization

Utilized Care Services	*Preferred Services of*		*Total*
	Missionary hospital	*Non-missionary hospital*	
Inside Manipur	2	27	
Outside Manipur	2	39	
Total	**4**	**66**	**70**

Source: Field Survey, 2003.

From this table we can see that the missionaries did not play an active role in informing the women in regard to their reproductive health (Table 4.13). In the Lamka town, the non-missionary sources like the health workers, doctors and health department advertisements, have disseminated information regarding their menstrual cycle and keeping clean during the period as well as informed them about the various RTI/STI and their causes and prevention on a wide scale to the women (Table 4.13).

Table 4.13: Knowledge about Reproductive Health

Information Pertaining to:	*Source of Information from the*		*Total*
	Missionaries	*Non-missionaries*	
Menstrual Cycle	7	33	
RTI/STI: Its causes	2	28	
Total	**9**	**61**	**70**

Source: Field Survey, 2003.

The Lamka women have derived more information pertaining to reprouctive health from the non-missionary sources. Majority of them have acquired information in regard to immunization during pregnancy (Table 4.14). Very few of them have received information about the identification of high risk pregnancy (Table 4.14). The advertisement placed by the health department about small family norm through posters, media and other means have gained access to the Lamka women (Table 4.14).

Table 4.14: Knowledge of Reproductive Health Programmes

Knowledge Pertaining to:	*Source of information from*		*Total*
	Missionaries	*Non-missionaries*	
Small Family Norm	0	19	
Ante-Natal Care	0	9	
Immunization during Pregnancy	2	32	
Identification of high risk pregnancy	0	8	
Total	**2**	**68**	**70**

Source: Field Survey, 2003.

The missionaries did not inform as well as made provision for the availability of contraceptives according to the Lamka town women. They opined that the missionaries were against birth control and informing the women in regard to the same would be blasphemous. The non-missionary sources provided all the information in relation to the contraceptives to the women of the town (Table 4.15) and a majority of the women have used the oral pills, next to it was the condom which was found to be easy in usage as well as availability. Very few of the women have gone in for abortion as compared to the women of Takvom village (Table 4.15).

Table 4.15: Utilization of Contraceptives

Type of Contraceptives Used	*Source of Supply from*		*Total*
	Missionary hospital	*Non-missionary hospital*	
Vasectomy	0	6	
Tubectomy	0	9	
Total Sterilization	0	5	
IUCD	0	5	
Oral Pills	0	27	
Condoms	0	12	
MTP	0	6	
Total	**0**	**70**	**70**

Source: Field Survey, 2003.

The women of Lamka town received the maximum information regarding cleanliness of the house from both the missionary and non-missionary (Table 4.16). The women of the town gave credit to the missionary for informing their parents about hygiene which then got passed on to them in the present times. Information regarding having a toilet instead of doing it in the open as well as proper storage of drinking water was all informed by the missionary. The non-missionaries also played a role in informing the women about hygiene (Table 4.16) but their first source of information was the missionaries.

Table 4.16: Awareness Regarding Hygiene

Awareness Regarding	*Source of Information from the*		*Total*
	Missionaries	*Non-missionaries*	
House Cleanliness	19	15	
Toilet Facility	11	9	
Storage of Drinking Water	9	7	
Total	**39**	**31**	**70**

Source: Field Survey, 2003.

The women of Lamka town are also meat lovers like the Takvom village women (Table 4.17). Meat forms an essential part of their diet. Information regarding non-vegetarian diet was acquired from the non-missionary sources (Table 4.17). The women also mentioned that they received information about the caloric intake of an individual from the doctors in the hospital and very

Table 4.17: Awareness Regarding Nutrition

Awareness in Terms of:	*Source of Information from*		*Total*
	Missionaries	*Non-missionaries*	
Caloric intake of an individual	3	24	
Non-vegetarian diet	6	30	
Follow of Food Routine	1	6	
Total	**10**	**60**	**70**

Source: Field Survey, 2003.

few of the women did not negate the role of the missionary in this regard (Table 4.17). The women also mentioned that they did not receive much information about following a proper food routine either from the missionary or the non-missionary sources (Table 4.17).

The above table shows that majority of the women in the Lamka town felt the missionaries involvement in spreading health awareness was minimal. However, according to them the missionaries did help spread information regarding good health and thereby ensuring that the tribal visited qualified doctors during ill-health instead of quacks. The women in Lamka preferred to go to the private clinics or the bigger hospital in the capital, Imphal. As for major illness such as cancer, heart problem, throat cancer, breast cancer etc. they would go to Vellore, Bombay or Delhi for their health check-up (Table 4.12). Majority of the women opined that the missionaries did not spread any awareness about reproductive health programmes (Table 4.14) instead, they were opposed to abortion and use of contraceptives (Table 4.15).

They were made aware about the RH programmes mainly through words of mouth as well as the various posters and advertisements taken out by the district hospitals in collaboration with the State Government.

The missionaries' involvement was acknowledged in spreading awareness about hygiene and nutrition (Table 4.16 and Table 4.17) they were now practicing hygienic living standards as compared to earlier times.

From Table 4.18, we can conclude that the missionaries have been instrumental in bringing about educational facilities in the town. Majority of the women felt that the missionaries have brought about a change in their attitude towards education (Table 4.18). Most of the women preferred to send their children to a missionary school because the facility when compared with a non-missionary school, is much better.

According to them in the non-missionary school although the teaching medium is English most of the teachers resort to the local dialect while teaching. The number of qualified teachers within the missionary school is also much more than the non-missionary

Table 4.18: Criteria for a School

Criteria for School	*School Preferred*		*Total*
	Missionary school	*Non-missionary school*	
English Medium	21	12	
Qualified Teachers	15	4	
Quality of Teaching	15	3	
Total	**51**	**19**	**70**

Source: Field Survey, 2003.

school where the school teachers are recruited mostly in terms of face value by the concerned principal (Table 4.18). Many of the women also feel that the quality of education is the best in the missionary school because the school does not offer much holidays and do not close down unnecesarily like the non-missionary school, private and government.

The Adolescent Group

Adolescence is a period of transition from childhood to adulthood. It is the period of life between the ages of 10-19 yrs. Health problems of adolescents are very different from those of younger children and older adults. Due to lack of accurate information, adolescents are prone to various behavioural and reproductive health problems.

Physical and Physiological Changes During Adolescence

Puberty in Girls

During puberty in females, they subjected to the appearance of hair in the pubic area, and breast begins to grow. Other changes include accelerated growth and development of genital organs. Menarche is the onset of first menstruation that occurs in girls. There are variations in the age at which menarche occurs.

Puberty in Boys

Puberty in boys usually appears later than girls. It may begin with a change in the voice, growth of hair in the chin, under arms, face, chest, and pubic region. Development/enlargement of external genitals also takes place and sperms production starts.

For the porpose of collecting information about puberty and adolescent health the researcher interviewed 65 adolescent (both boys and girls) within the age group of 16 to 18 years. This adolescent group was from different discipline.

Most of the adolescent interviewed had good knowledge regarding adolescent health. However, many of them were unable to clearly define what is meant by the term "puberty" but could at the same time inform the researcher about the physical changes which both the boys and girls undergo as they reach puberty. All the girls interviewed mentioned that as the boys reach puberty their voice cracks and that their moustaches develop moreover, in some cases their pimples also comes out. Their main source of information was the school and precisely the science class. They also mentioned that their knowledge about the physical changes is more deepened because of the conversation they have about boys among their friends circle. Similarly, when enquired about the girls physical changes with the onset of puberty. Most of the boys interviewed were able to inform the researcher about the physical changes which a girl undergoes once she reaches puberty. Some of boys were a bit hesitant to answer the question put forward to them.

Out of the total girls interviewed, many of them were well informed in advance about the menstrual cycle. Their mother as well as from the school peer group gave this information to them if anyone starts to menstruate. Only some of the girls did not have any information about the menstrual cycle but slowly became aware of it once they started menstruating. Moreover the girls informed the researcher that their menstrual cycle was regular and on being asked what would be the reason if irrigularity persists then many of them said that as one gets older the cycle tends to change and it is a normal process however rest of the girls opined that irregularity occurs mainly due to the poor health of the female. None of them related irregularity with being pregnant. Nevertheless, they mentioned that if the cycle stops for more than a month and that they have involved themselves in a physical relation, and then it would definitely mean that they are pregnant.

Majority of the girls use sanitary napkins. None of them were found to be using cloths. As for the sanitary napkins, they use approximately 8 to 10 pads every cycle and these pads after being used are wrapped in a paper and thrown in the dustbin. The choice of sanitary napkins for the girls ranges from *Whisper* to *She* to *Kotex* to *Stayfree,* which meant that all types of sanitary napkins are available to them. The first got information about sanitary napkins from the television advertisement as well as from their friends who study out of town. The choices for sanitary napkins also depend upon the buying capacity of the girls and their family.

Regarding their participation in the church services most of the girls informed the researcher that during menstrual cycle their life does not stop in fact, they continue with their normal tasks and do not keep themselves in isolation. However, only few of them out of the total 45 girls interviewed mentioned that they keep away from the religious activities. When asked the reason, they informed the researcher that the flow is heavy and so most of the time they are scared that it would stain their dress. Only due to the fear of being embarrassed they do not attend the church services.

Out of the total 65 adolescent interviewed, most knew about reproductive organs but they could not specify the organs and their functions. Only a very few of them knew the functions of the reproductive organs by virtue of being in the science stream. Many of the adolescent have not heard of the reproductive ill health problems but the rest of them have heard about the reproductive ill health problems. Howe0ver, none of the 65 adolescent interviewed have not experienced any of the reproductive ill health problems.

All of them have heard about AIDs/HIV and they were well informed about the causative as well as the preventive method. They acquired their information from the school as well as the awareness campaign that is organized at least once in a month in

Lamka due to the reason that Lamka has a high percentage of infected persons with HIV/AIDS. All the more many of their friends have indulged themselves in the substance abuse and few of them have even died due to overdose of such drugs. Both the adolescent boys and girls have heard about the reproductive health programmes mainly through the posters that are being set up in and around the town. This is to say that their information about the reproductive health programme has been generated mainly from the family welfare programme campaign.

Majority of the adolescent respondents were aware about the different types of contraceptives that are available. Their source of information ranged from friends to doctors to the advertisements. Very few of them completely denied having heard about contraceptives. Here, the bias of the researcher is reflected as she feels that the respondents who claim not to have any information about the contraceptives are not being truthful because they are of the opinion that both girls and boys having information about the different types of contraceptives are of a dubious character.

Among the 65 adolescent respondents, few of them were of the opinion that sex education should not be imparted in the school, as it would give the students a "knowledge" licence to have physical relations with the opposite sex.

The more they are unaware of the precautions they are afraid of the repercussions and would hence avoid such relations. However, majority of them put forward that once a person is matured enough to understand what he/she wants then it is their choice however, in order to prevent them from any kind of unwanted pregnancies and sexually transmitted diseases it is important to inform them about the various precautions they should undertake if they are entering into a physical relations with the opposite sex.

Apart from this, majority of them felt that career counselling and family values should also be covered whereby children will learn to respect their parents and parents in turn love their children.

Ephesians 6:1-4 "Children, obey your parents in the lord, foe this is right. Honour your father and mother, which is the first commandment with a promise that, it may go well with you and that you may enjoy long life on the earth. Fathers, do not exasperate your children; instead, bring them up in the training and instructions of the lord".

Many of the adolescent respondents were of the notion that the media can definitely play a major role in disseminating information about reproduction and sexuality as it will be more receptive, for the people because not everyone is educated and therefore, media in the form of the local dialect will act as a good medium of informing the people and will be able to influence the mindset of the people.

Again, the adolescent group was of the opinion that the teachers can also help in disseminating information regarding reproductive health and sexuality because teachers are experienced as well as more competent to inform the students. Moreover, the students believe the teachers look upon them and whatever they say is generally not questioned. Peer groups also influence one another and it also helps in spreading such information, as there are no inhibitions among each other. Things are talked openly among the peers group. The adolescent group interviewed had good knowledge about the importance of good education and the changes it can bring about. Although, they all belong to the tribal population it was evident from the conversation that they are all trying to carve a niche for themselves and are no longer dependent on living life in the fast lane.

The following tables inform us about the *female adolescents* and their access to information and knowledge regarding the different aspects of health and health care and whether there has been an involvement of the missionaries in this regard.

In the following tables the *Missionary sources* includes: the local pastor, Church youth group, Church women's group, Church literature.

The *non-missionary sources* includes: the government health workers, doctors and nurses, NGOs working in the specific field, volunteers of diffeent NGOs and peer groups.

Table 4.19 shows that there is more of a non-missionary intervention in regard to informing the adolescent about puberty.

According to the females interviewed they informed the researcher that they received information pertaining to puberty from their schools and the physical changes in boys was known to them through observation and discussion with peer groups and that there was not much of missionary intervention (Table 4.19).

Table 4.19: Female Adolescents' Opinion Knowledge about Puberty

Knowledge about	*Source of information*		*Total*
	Missionary	*Non-missionary*	
Puberty	5	21	
Physical changes in boys	0	19	
Total	**5**	**40**	**45**

Source: Field Survey, 2003.

The female adolescents were very clear as to where they want to go whenever they experienced any ill-health. Out of the total female adolescent interviewed not many of them sought care from the missionary run hospital during ill-health (Table 4.20) as compared to those who sought care from the non-missionary hospital. Typhoid was the ill-health least experienced by the adolescent and viral fever was the most common ill-health experienced by the female adolescent in majority (Table 4.20).

Table 4.20: Female Adolescents and their Health Seeking Services

Type of Ill-health	*Care Sought from*		*Total*
Experienced	*Missionary hospital*	*Non-missionary hospital*	
Malaria	1	9	
Diarrhea	0	10	
Viral Fever	0	13	
Typhoid	1	4	
Jaundice	0	7	
Total	**2**	**43**	**45**

Source: Field Survey, 2003.

Whenver the female adolescents experienced any of the ill-health (Table 4.20), they preferred to go to the non-missionary hospital (Table 4.21). Majority of the female adolescent emphasized that they would go outside Manipur in case of severe problems (Table 4.21). Not many prefer to seek care services within Manipur as they feel that the doctors would not be qualified. More so, the facilities available outside would be more advanced and state-of-the-art. In Manipur, though many private hospital have come up in the recent years it does not provide proper satisfaction to the care seekers.

Table 4.21: Female Adolescents and Their Care Services Utilization

Utilized Care Services	*Preferred Services of*		*Total*
	Missionary hospital	*Non-missionary hospital*	
Inside Manipur	2	13	
Outside Manipur	2	28	
Total	**4**	**41**	**45**

Source: Field Survey, 2003.

The female adolescents opined that they did not receive any information regarding reproductive health from the missionaries, the only information the missionaries gave was pertaining to the cleanliness pattern during the menstrual cycle (Table 4.22). Most of their information was collected from the non-missionary sources like, schools and peer groups. The female emphasized that they received prior information regarding their menstrual cycle from their mothers and through their friends who already expereinced menstrual cycle (Table 4.22).

Regarding the RTI/STI, its causes and prevention the female adolescent informed the researcher that they got the information from non-missionary sources like the nurses and the health workers who would come to their schools. Information regarding usage of sanitary napkins was all acquired from the media in particular television and friends as well as by word of mouth regarding the best sanitary napkins (Table 4.22).

Table 4.22: Female Adolescents and their Knowledge about Reproductive Health

Information Pertaining to:	*Source of Information from*		*Total*
	Missionaries	*Non-missionaries*	
Menstrual Cycle	0	12	
Usage of Sanitary Napkins	1	8	
Drying of menstrual cloth	0	2	
Cleanliness during Cycle	5	6	
RTI/STI: Its causes and Prevention	1	10	
Total	**7**	**38**	**45**

Source: Field Survey, 2003.

The female adolescents received the maximum information regarding small family norm and their source of information was mainly the non-missionary sources, advertisement (Table 4.23). They also mentioned that they prefer to have a small family when they get married as they would like to provide all the necessity to their children.

Table 4.23: Female Adolescents' Knowledge of Reproductive Health Programmes

Knowledge Pertaining to:	*Source of information from*		*Total*
	Missionaries	*Non-missionaries*	
Small Family Norm	0	31	
Anti-Natal Care	0	1	
Immunization during Pregnancy	2	11	
Identification of high risk pregnancy	0	0	
Total	**2**	**43**	**45**

Source: Field Survey, 2003.

None of them had received information regarding the identification of high risk pregnancy (Table 4.23). Few of the female adolescents have informed the researcher that they have heard about the importance of getting proper immunization during pregnancy but their source of information was mostly the non-missionary source (Table 4.23).

Majority of the female adolescents had information about contraceptives and this information was made available to them by the non-missionary sources like schools, hospitals, advertisement etc. They opined that they received no information regarding contraceptives from the missionary sources (Table 4.24).

Table 4.24: Female Adolescents and Their Knowledge about Contraceptives

Type of Contraceptives	*Source of Supply from*		*Total*
	Missionary hospital	*Non-missionary hospital*	
Vasectomy	0	1	
Tubectomy	0	3	
Total Sterilization	0	1	
IUCD	0	2	
Oral Pills	0	12	
Condoms	0	12	
MTP	0	14	
Total	**0**	**45**	**45**

Source: Field Survey, 2003.

Many of the female adolescents have the knowledge about oral pills as well as contraceptives; this information was shared among the peer groups. Majority of them have good information about abortion and till what period it is safe to go in for abortion (Table 4.24).

The female adolescents did not have much information regarding the other contraceptives method like vasectomy, tubectomy, total sterilization and IUCD (Table 4.24).

The female adolescents mentioned that both the missionary and the non-missionary have helped to spread the information about keeping a house clean (Table 4.25). They were not very sure regarding the information pertaining to the toilet facility but few did acknowledge that the missionary brought about awareness regarding having a toilet facility. Of the total female adolescents interviewed most of them felt that the information pertaining the need to store drinking water was put forward by the non-missionary sources (Table 4.25).

Table 4.25: Female Adolescents and Their Awareness Regarding Hygiene

Awareness Regarding	*Source of Information from the*		*Total*
	Missionaries	*Non-missionaries*	
House Cleanliness	12	17	
Toilet Facility	2	4	
Storage of Drinking Water	3	7	
Total	**17**	**28**	**45**

Source: Field Survey, 2003.

The female adolescents stressed that the people love meat in the district and its forms an integral part of their diet. However, the consumption of non-vegetarian food during meals was not specified by the missionaries as compared to the non-missionaries (Table 4.26). They further mentioned that the information they have regarding the caloric intake of an individual was not passed on from the missionaries but this information was given to them by their school (Table 4.26). They even informed the researcher that the knowledge about following of a food routine was not specified by the missionaries as much as the non-missionaries (Table 4.26).

Table 4.26: Female Adolescents and Their Knowledge Regarding Nutrition

Knowledge in Terms of:	*Source of Information from*		*Total*
	Missionaries	*Non-missionaries*	
Caloric intake of an individual	0	13	
Non-vegetarian diet	3	22	
Follow of Food Routine	1	6	
Total	**4**	**41**	**45**

Source: Field Survey, 2003.

The females adolescents voted highly in favour of a missionary run school in order to have good education (Table 4.27). They were of the opinion that the missionary run educational institutes had more qualified teachers than the non-missionary schools because of which the quality of teaching is also better and enables the students to grasp more information as compared to the non-missionary school whose teachers often take classes in their local dialect which does not leave much scope for the students to understand English properly (Table 4.27). They also prefer going to the missionary schools because it keeps them involve in different kinds of extra-curricular activities such as career counselling, personality trainings and that they also take Family Life Education classes.

Table 4.27: Female Adolescents Criteria for a School

Criteria for School	*School Preferred*		*Total*
	Missionary school	*Non-missionary school*	
English Medium	13	1	
Qualified Teachers	11	3	
Quality of teaching	12	5	
Total	**36**	**9**	**45**

Source: Field Survey, 2003.

The researcher was also informed that the Family Life Education commonly known as Moral Science class was started by the missionary school and gradually it was adopted by the non-missionary school as it helped the students to develop better understanding about their life grow as a better human being.

Hence, one can say that the adolescents in contrast to the women of both Takvom village and Lamka town felt that the missionaries were not involved in the provision of health care (Tables 4.3 and 4.11). Very few of them did not rule out the Missionaries involvement. The adolescents were of the opinion that all the information about health have been provided to them by the doctors and the government. Schools have also disseminated information in regards to menstrual health (Table 4.22) and hygiene (Table 4.25) apart from the posters and drawing which carries messages like "birth by choice not by chance".

Moreover, the adolescents informed the researcher that if they ever had to consult a doctor regarding their illness or their family members, then they would approach a private practitioner rather than a government one as doctors who are practicing privately seem to be more dedicated when compared with the government doctors who do not even give a patient hearing to the health problems of the people who come for check-up (Table 4.21). They are also willing to spend a huge amount of money for care services as long as they are satisfied with the kind of services provided.

The following tables inform us about the *male adolescents* and their access to information and knowledge regarding the different aspects of health and health care and whether there has been an involvement of the missionaries in this regard.

In the following tables the *Missionary sources* includes: the local pastor, Church youth group, Church women's group, Church literature.

The *non-missionary sources* includes: the government health workers, doctors and nurses, NGOs working in the specific field, volunteers of different NGOs and peer groups.

The adolescent boys completely denied the involvement of the missionary regarding their knowledge about the physical changes in the females (Table 4.28). They specified that they knew about it from their own observation, their talks with their peer groups as well as from their school in their biology classes. They even mentioned that their knowledge about puberty was collected from their classes and not necessarily informed to them by the missionaries (Table 4.28).

Table 4.28: Male Adolescents and Their Knowledge about Puberty

Knowledge about	*Source of information*		*Total*
	Missionary	*Non-missionary*	
Puberty	2	11	
Physical changes in boys	0	7	
Total	**2**	**18**	**20**

Source: Field Survey, 2003.

Like the female adolescents (Table 4.20), the male Adolescents also sought care for any ill-health experienced from the non-missionary hospital. Most of the boys interviewed mentioned that they have had diarrhea (Table 4.29) and few of them have experienced malaria as well as jaundice. The boys further informed the researcher that the type of illness which they mostly experience was seasonal.

Table 4.29: Male Adolescents and Their Health Seeking Services

Type of Ill-health	*Care Sought from*		*Total*
Experienced	*Missionary hospital*	*Non-missionary hospital*	
Malaria	1	2	
Diarrhea	0	7	
Viral Fever	0	5	
Typhoid	0	3	
Jaundice	0	2	
Total	**1**	**19**	**20**

Source: Field Survey, 2003.

The male adolescent mentioned that for the utilization of the care services they prefer going to the non-missionary run health centres such as the private clinics. They even mentioned that if need arises they would go and seek care outside Manipur (Table 4.30) as the facilities would be much better than the ones within Manipur. Very few of them did not mind going to the missionary run health centres within and outside Manipur as long as they got good treatment (Table 4.30).

Table 4.30: Male Adolescents and Their Care Services Utilization

Utilized Care	*Preferred Services of*		*Total*
Services	*Missionary hospital*	*Non-missionary hospital*	
Inside Manipur	2	5	
Outside Manipur	2	11	
Total	**4**	**16**	**20**

Source: Field Survey, 2003.

According to the male adolescents the missionary were not involved in spreading information regarding the different types of contraceptives (Table 4.31). The adolescent boys' knowledge pertaining to contraceptives was derived from non-missionary sources mainly their peer groups and through the advertisement taken out by the health department. Many of them were aware about condoms as well as oral pills (Table 4.31). None of them have ever utilized even one of the contraceptives but they have heard about it only. They had the least information about vasectomy, tubectomy, total sterilization and IUCD as well.

Table 4.31: Male Adolescents and Their Knowledge about Contraceptives

Type of Contraceptives	*Source of Supply from*		*Total*
	Missionary hospital	*Non-missionary hospital*	
Vasectomy	0	1	
Tubectomy	0	1	
Total Sterilization	0	1	
IUCD	0	1	
Oral Pills	0	5	
Condoms	0	8	
MTP	0	3	
Total	**0**	**20**	**20**

Source: Field Survey, 2003.

The adolescent boys felt that the missionary as well as the non-missionaries have been active in spreading information regarding cleanliness (Table 4.32). Although majority of them

Table 4.32: Male Adolescents and Their Awareness Regarding Hygiene

Awareness Regarding	*Source of Information from the*		*Total*
	Missionaries	*Non-missionaries*	
House Cleanliness	3	8	
Toilet Facility	1	3	
Storage of Drinking Water	1	4	
Total	**5**	**15**	**20**

Source: Field Survey, 2003.

mentioned that the non-missionaries involvement in bringing about awareness regarding hygiene was more, they did not completely negate the missionaries' role also. Information about construction of toilet was also informed by the missionaries (Table 4.32) as well as the proper storage of drinking water.

The adolescent boys did not acknowledge the involvement of the missionaries in bringing about awareness regarding nutrition (Table 4.33). They stressed that the non-missionary sources like, the government and health workers, were entirely responsible for developing awareness among the people in regard to proper nutrition. They gave credits to them for informing the people about the caloric intake of an individual and also the need to follow a balance food routine (Table 4.33).

Table 4.33: Male Adolescents and Their Knowledge Regarding Nutrition

Knowledge in Terms of:	*Source of Information from*		*Total*
	Missionaries	*Non-missionaries*	
Caloric intake of an individual	0	9	
Non-vegetarian diet	0	8	
Follow of Food Routine	0	3	
Total	**0**	**20**	**20**

Source: Field Survey, 2003.

The missionary run educational institutes is the most popular among the adolescent boys (Table 4.34). According to them, the missionary school provides the best platform to attain good education as the teachers are qualified as well as the teaching methods used by the school is very efficient (Table 4.34).

The missionaries' schools also have periods whereby they give career counselling, take sessions on sex education as well as hold classes for Family Life Education unlike the non-missionary schools. The boys even mentioned that the non-missionary schools are also English medium but the English language is not used most of the times even by the teachers themselves (Table 4.34).

Table 4.34: Male Adolescents' Criteria for a School

Criteria for School	*School preferred*		*Total*
	Missionary	*Non-missionary*	
English Medium	9	1	
Qualified Teachers	4	1	
Quality of teaching	4	1	
Total	**17**	**3**	**20**

Source: Field Survey, 2003.

Thus, from the above tables it is reflected that the adolescent boys feel that the missionaries' involvement in their health (Table 4.29), hygiene (Table 4.32), nutrition (Table 4.33) etc. is not much however they do not completely deny their involvement.

Nevertheless, the missionaries' involvement in the education has been acknowledged on a large scale (Table 4.34). Most of the adolescent boys interviewed were studying in a missionary run schools. They are of the opinion that the missionaries have ushered in the desire to know more and the importance of education at every stage of life.

Takvom Village Women, Lamka Town Women and the Adolescent Group: An Analysis

Regarding health care awareness among the Takvom village women it has been found that they have a better knowledge about viral fever with or without the help of the missionaries. They have the least awareness about typhoid.

Similarly in the Lamka town the women have better awareness regarding the cause and prevention of viral fever. This could cause viral fever is more dominant as compared to the other ill-health.

The adolescent group also mentioned that they have more information about the viral fever and the least information about typhoid. Though they did not completely deny the involvement of the missionaries in the spread of this knowledge, very few of them acknowledged the missionaries role in spreading awareness about the various ill-health.

The reproductive health programme have not been touched by the missionaries nevertheless, information regarding the immunization during pregnancy have been informed by the missionaries in the village whenever the case of pregnancy was present in the village. Thus, information on a large scale about the reproductive health has been acquired from the district hospitals and the health workers who come to the village once in a while.

The maximum information given by the health workers was pertaining to the immunization during pregnancy and not much information was being given about the ante-natal care. Identification of high risk pregnancy was not done by the health workers but only by the doctors that too, when a visit to the district hospital was made. There was no information pertaining to high risk pregnancy. Apart from this, information was also derived from the various posters which are seen while travelling in and around the district. For the Lamka women information regarding reproductive health has also been passed on to them from the health workers and not the missionaries. The nurses in the hospitals also spread about the programmes by word of mouth. The number of women having access to ante-natal care is more than the Takvom village women. A large proportion of the Lamka town women have acquired information regarding the reproductive health programmes.

The adolescent group in particular the females have acquired more information regarding the cleanliness pattern during the menstrual cycle and the usage of sanitary napkins was derived from their peer groups, by their respective schools as well as the advertisement. The female adolescents are of the opinion that information regarding the menstrual cycle have not been given to them by the missionaries.

There are also some similarities between the Takvom village women and the Lamka town women in regards to their information about the various contraceptives. They have more information about oral pills and condoms and many of the women interviewed in both the areas mentioned having used the oral pills and the condoms. Medical termination of pregnancy (MTP) was generally not utilized by the women of both the study areas. They feel that MTP was against their moral upbringing and that they have no right to kill an urborn child which have been the creation of God.

The adolescent group in Churachandpur district comprising both the Takvom village and the Lamka town also have more information regarding the oral pills and the condom. They also have knowledge about the MTP which is known as abortion. Among the male adolescent very few mentioned that they would go in for total sterilization.

Women of Takvom village live in houses made of bamboo but are nevertheless able to keep their houses clean. The Lamka town women are living in *pucca* houses and they are also able to maintain their houses in a proper manner. The missionaries have been able to bring about cleanliness and hygiene among the people and these have helped the people to maintain a clean surrounding with their home.

The women of Takvom village still have toilets which are not properly constructed, they are more like a deep hole that has been dugged for the purpose. In Lamka town, the women feel that the information regarding toilet facility has not been spread by the missionaries.

The toilets in Lamka town have now been properly constructed. The Lamka town people prefer the Indian style toilet than the English style.

Being a tribal population many of the people are non-vegetarian. Meat forms a basic diet during meals. Green leafy vegetables which are mainly boiled are also taken by the women in large numbers. The food habit of both Lamka town and the Takvom village inhabitants are similar. There is no difference in the preference of their eating habit. The only difference which one can talk about is the method of cooking. The Lamka town use gas cylinders for cooking whereas the Takvom villagers still use stove for cooking.

Information regarding seeking health care services inside Manipur was much lesser as compared to the people who would go outside Manipur for health check-up. The women of Lamka town mentioned that they would probably go outside Manipur if they were suffering from any health problems.

However, the women of the Takvom village informed the researcher that they would go to the district hospital in Lamka town for their care seeking and the furthest they would go for attaining care services would be the capital, Imphal.

The adolescent group mentioned that for their health care in regard to major ill-health they do not rely upon the doctors in the district though they may be well-qualified but they would prefer to go outside Manipur as the facilities would be more and that there would be more specialized doctors.

In relation to the educational facilities the adolescent groups have voted in support of the missionaries. Majority of them are of the opinion that the missionaries have started the pioneering work of spreading the importance of education.

The adolescent group interviewed, opined that the missionaries' schools are the best in the district and that they would also want their children to study in the missionaries' school itself. Their main reason for supporting the missionaries' schools is due to the fact that the quality of education is better than any other schools and that the missionaries' schools also have provision of Family Life Education which enable an adolescent to grow up to be a responsible human being.

The women of Takvom village and the Lamka town share a certain level of similarities in terms of their information about the various fields such as ill-health, reproductive health programmes, contraceptives, information regarding hygiene and nutrition, as well as services to be accessed during ill-health. They however acknowledged the involvement of the missionaries in all the fields as compared to the present adolescent group who did not want to give credit to the missionaries nevertheless very few of them did acknowledged the missionaries for bringing about a transformation among the Paite tribe from being a tribal group to a more civilized group.

Dialogue with the Elder

Reverend Siamkung was born in 1920 and got married in 1944. His third wife passed away on April 2004.

The researcher interviewed him in order to know how the Paite tribal people lived during the early period before the advent of missionaries as well as education. In more ways, he was interviewed to understand the differences that exist during the earlier times and now.

About the Meeting

He informed the worker that Christianity entered Churachandpur district on the *7th of May 1910* and that the North-East India General Mission (NEIG) started it. His parents became the first Evengelist when Evengelical mission was discovered in the state of Mizoram. His father's name is Tualthang and mother's name is Chalruali. The following is an abstract of the interview held with him.

When asked about the lifestyle of the people in the society before and after the spread of education and Christianity, Rev. Siamkung informed the researcher that there has been great development in Lamka as compared to the earlier years. People have progressed from a nomadic lifestyle to a westernized lifestyle. Till Christianity came to the people, every tribe was self-sufficient and idol worship was done by all the different tribes.

There were no qualified doctors and the only doctors available were the "*siampu*" (local doctor) apart from the army and the missionary's doctors. Many people would suffer from illness but that time the ill causing factor was not known. Moreover there was no specific name for the illness. "Name would be given according to the spirit that they believed have bitten the ill person.

There was only one hospital for the entire Churachandpur and for medicines they had to travel to Gauhati or Shillong. Slowly, there was a drift away from the *"siampu"* but the *siampu* were not completely ignored. *"Ki-thoih"* (sacrifice) performed for any illness, *i.e.* asking the spirits for favour. If the spirit returns the favour, then they consider the illness to be cured. There is no concept of medicines" (Luaizakham, 1991, 19).

The people would depend upon the spring water or pond for drinking and other purposes. They would never boil water before drinking. *"Tui-thei"* (use to store water) is made out of the bamboo tree.

There was no notion of hygiene among the population. He told the researcher that the people were not accustomed to taking bath and the dress that they wear would be changed only when it tears off or during seasonal celebrations.

The people would use *"Meleng"*, (fruit of a tree) to wash clothes with. Food was eaten on a banana leave but slowly plates became a common sight but then also these plates were not washed but licked by the dogs and then re-used for eating purposes. Sometimes the whole family would even eat out of the same plate that was large in size.

Since there was no toilet, everyone do it in the open and the pigs would be called and then they would feed upon it. To clean themselves, the people use a stick instead of water.

Electric supply in Lamka is not frequent but the situation now is better than before when there was no electricity and the people depended upon natural light or used *"Meilah"* which would burn for more than 2 to 3 hours. *"Meisel"* was also used but this would burn for a very short time. Then, as the missionaries started to settle in the town there was the use of oil lamps, torch etc. This was again used by the economically better-off people. He informed the worker that those who could afford the torchlight were looked up as a rich man.

Barter system was very prominent during those times. People would generally exchange cooked vegetables with their neighbours. This shows that solidarity was prevalent and there would be no conflict in the name of faith, tribe, status etc. The value of money was a lot because there was not much money in the district. People could go to Imphal with even one *dere* (traditional term for one anna).

When the foreign missionaries entered Manipur, the people looked upon them with awe and whatever they did was imitated as well as whatever they told the villagers were listened to and followed. There was no concept of wrong to whatever they said. Before the missionaries started preaching the word of God, incest was prevalent on a large scale.

He further mentioned that the missionaries have brought about a lot of changes in the society and that people have been able to know what is going in other society through the means of education spread by the missionaries.

Moreover, almost half the adolescent population in Churachandpur have gone outside in search of better educational facilities in different parts of the country.

At the same time he opined that the different missionaries who have visited Churachandpur have also caused the breaking up of a close knit society and giving rise to a number of churches based on different faith.

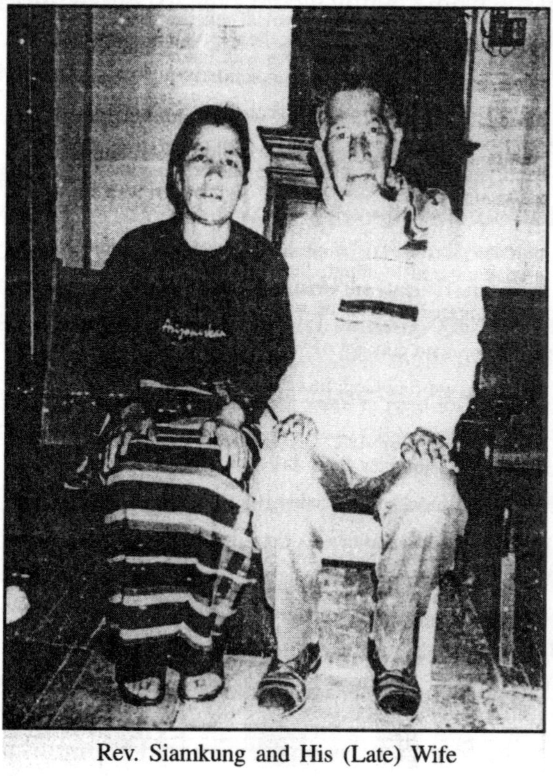

Rev. Siamkung and His (Late) Wife

Meeting with the District Family Welfare Officer

The Family Welfare Office is located in the District Hospital, Lamka. Many people go to the District Hospital for seeking care facility. The following is an extract of interview with the District Family Welfare Officer (DFWO).

Dr. Thangkhenkham Hartlang is the District Family Welfare Officer. In addition to this he is also the RCH Programme Officer of the district. He joined the district hospital as a DFWO on October 15th, 1997. In the Churachandpur District Reproductive Child Health Programme was initiated since 2000. Till date there are 15 RCH centres in the district. The RCH programme relates to the current policy of the target free approach at the grassroots level under the new reproductive and child health initiative of the Government of India.

According to Dr. Hartlang 72 per cent of the women in the district seek care regarding RCH in the district hospital. This has been a recent development as compared to the earlier times when the women were not comfortable in consulting the doctor for reproduction related care. As of now there is a gynaecological OPD as well as a STD clinic in the district hospital.

He further mentioned that contraceptives such as Copper-T, condom and contraceptive pills are supplied free of cost by the Urban Family Welfare Centre. However during July and August 2003, there was no supply of Copper-T, he opined that the supply at the state level was stopped and consequently the district supply also suffered.

He even informed the researcher that in the Post-Partum centre, Family Planning advice is given as well as the operation is undertaken. This has helped many couples to choose their contraceptive method and take decision accordingly. The hospital records show that the temporary methods of birth control are more prevalent.

In 1980s Immunization was started in the district and a large number of expecting mother as well as the ones with infants immunized themselves. For the year 2003-04, the Intensified Pulse

Polio Immunization (IPPI) was started under the District Family Welfare Unit.

Table 4.35: The Following Hospital Records show that the Temporary Method of Birth Control is more Prevalent

Family Planning Activities	*2000-01*	*2001-02*	*2002-03*
Vasectomy	79	0	8
Tubectomy	252	277	242
Total Sterilization	331	277	250
IUCD	386	328	393
Oral Pills User	400	—	920
Condoms	19930	18051	11162
MTP	628	723	871

Source: Family Welfare Programme and RCH Project Records.

Dr. Hartlang emphasized that Information Education and Communication (IEC) activities are an integral part of the RCH programme. Thus, in order to increase the awareness among the people big board, poster, banners etc. with RCH messages were put up within the district headquarters area and the nearby villages. According to him this has led to an increased awareness about the Family Planning Programmes.

5

Summary, Findings and Conclusion

Summary

Before beginning the research work, the researcher looked up the census data in relation to the state of Manipur in order to have an overall knowledge about the study area. The findings from the census data is as follows:

Churachandpur is popularly known as Lamka district.

The total population of Manipur is 23,88,634: male = 12,07,338 and females = 11,81,296 (2001 census). The total population of Churachandpur district is 2,28,707: males = 1,14,740 and females = 1,13,967 (2001 census). Takvom village fall within the district and has a population of about 700. There is about 70 households within the Takvom village.

The sex ratio of Manipur is 978 per 1000 males (2001 census). The sex ratio of Churachandpur district is 993 per 1000 males (2001 census).

The literacy rate of Manipur is 69.87 per cent. Males = 77.87 per cent and females = 59.70 per cent (2001 census). The literacy rate of Churachandpur district is 74.67 per cent. Males = 84.98 per cent and females = 64.40 per cent (2001 census). Takvom village literacy rate is not available in the census.

Christianity entered Manipur in the 20th century. Christianity entered the Churachandpur district on the 8th of May, 1910. Before Christianity entered the tribals' life they practiced *Ki-thoih,* popularly known as sacrifice for any ill-health within the family members. *Meilah* was used during the night time before the arrival of petromax (kerosene stove). *Dere* was the term given to one anna.

For problems regarding vaginal irritation the elder women of both the Takvom village and the Lamka town used *tangal* (cooking soda).

The Reproductive Child Health Programme was initiated in the district in the year 2000.

Lamka town have a better literacy rate as compared to Takvom village due to the fact that the number of both missionary (convent) schools as well as private and government schools is more in the town. The village of Takvom does not have any proper school and the children are not enrolled in the school. There is only one junior high school till class 8 which is under the zonal education officer. The children of Takvom village who want to study further have settled in Lamka town and are pursuing their education.

There has, however, been a rise in the educational status of the district due to the effort of the missionaries who first came to the district on the 7th of May, 1910. With the rise in education, development gradually progressed. In the present times the living standard of the Lamka town have seen a considerable increase, however, the living standard of the Takvom village have not seen any improvement. There has been on the contrary, an increase in the numbers of people who have migrated from the village in search of better living condition and employment.

Not only Paites but also people from West Bengal to Bihar have settled in the district and one can see the inter-mingling of people not only from Manipur but from all over the country, irrespective of belonging to different region and religion. There have, however, been few incidents of accidents in the district but it does not disrupt the peaceful environment which exists in the district. People from the Takvom village have also migrated to the district in search of better living conditions as well as for employment.

Many shops in the district have enabled people from the rural areas to gain employment. People are not only employed in government offices but there are others who have also opened shops such as electronic showroom, groceries store, confectionaries/ bakery stores and even restraurants. Most of the shops and restaurants are owned by the north Indians who have settled in the district and very few of the shops are owned by the people of Lamka. The people of Takvom do not own any of the shops in the district but some of them are employed in the shops.

The state of politics in the area have also seen a rise in the number of educated youths wanting to join politics in order to work for the betterment of the people. The youths have acquired education from within the district and even outside the district. The youths are from both Lamka town and the Takvom village. The majority of the youths joining politics are from Lamka town and very few from the Takvom village.

Education in the area is one of the major factors which have resulted in the outsourcing of many adolescent youths. Parents, rich or poor, sent their children to places like Delhi, Calcutta, Madras, Mumbai and near home like Nagaland, Shillong, and Gauhati to attain the best possible educational facilities. Many of the adolescent who have studied outside Manipur have done well in their professional life.

The number of people from Manipur who are in the high government services is on the rise, doctors and engineers are also on the rise as compared to the earlier times. Approximately about 18 per cent of the students' population from Churachandpur district are pursuing their B.A., M.A., M.Phil and Ph.D. from Jawaharlal Nehru University. With a rise in the educational status of the Paite people, information about the different aspects of life has also seen an improvement. Information, from education to health to living standards has percolated down even to the most rural areas.

The researcher in particular, has aimed to study the awareness of the Paite women regarding their health status. The study has enabled the researcher to acquire information about the Paite women health status. She has found out that the Paite women in both the Takvom village and the Lamka town have awareness regarding their health status as well as utilization of care services during ill-health moreover, the need to keep good health have gained importance as of now in comparison to the earlier times when seeking care for ill-health was limited till one could not go to the fields.

Health information particularly among the women in the Lamka town and the Takvom village has also increased. This could be because of the foundation laid by the missionaries who came to Churachandpur district which then slowly gained momentum.

A more civilized lifestyle/means of living have been in practiced since the arrival of the missionaries. The change in the lifestyle came about due to the various activities carried on by the missionaries.

Many women in the district have gained access to information regarding their reproductive health. The causes and prevention of many reproductive health problems have been disseminated by the health officials to the women and this information have also reached even the remotest village in the district. Women come to seek care for different types of ill-health from the district hospitals or certified doctors within Manipur but, majority would prefer to go outside Manipur for seeking care services for the different types of ill-health.

In contrast to the women of both the study areas, the adolescent groups have acquired information regarding the reproductive health and other issues mainly from their schools. As of the present times their source of information have become very wide they no longer rely only on one source but counter examine the variety of sources available to them. These sources include, newspaper, magazine, internet, peer groups etc.

The study have been undertaken by the researcher in order to examine whether there have been an improvement among the Paite women awareness level after the advent of Christianity as well as the spread of education in the Churachandpur district of Manipur.

In order to acquire information regarding the health of the Paite women in the Takvom village and the Lamka town, the researcher used the interview schedule. In both the study areas, the researcher has used the grab sampling methods to identify the sample population. In addition to it in-dept interview with the key informants were alo held. Apart from these, secondary sources were also used.

Findings

The fieldwork in the study areas, *i.e.* Takvom village and Lamka town have enabled the researcher to develop a better understanting of both the study areas in terms of their health awareness. The findings of the researcher are as follows:

(a) Health Seeking Services

The women of both Takvom village and Lamka town have experienced ill-health such as malaria, diarrhea, viral fever, typhoid and jaundice (Table 4.3 and Table 4.11). Majority of the women in both the area have sought care for these ill-health from the non-missionary hospital, however, few of them have also sought care from the missionary hospital as well. Majority of the adolescent group also sought care from the non-missionary hospital (Table 4.20 and Table 4.29).

(b) Care Services Utilization

Few of the women in the Takvom village sought care from the missionary hospital within Manipur and out of the total women interviewed half of them preferred to go outside Manipur for seeking care services (Table 4.4). The Lamka town women also seek care from the missionary hospital but the number is much lesser as compared to those who seek care from the non-missionary hospital. More than half of the women interviewed in the town preferred to go outside Manipur for seeking care services (Table 4.13). Among the adolescent, majority of them preferred to go for seeking care outside Manipur, only few of the adolescent sought care from the missionary sources within Manipur as compared to the majority who seek care from the non-missionary hospital (Table 4.21 and Table 4.30).

(c) Knowledge about Reproductive Helath

Majority of the Takvom village women have acquired information pertaining to the menstrual cycle and about RTI/STI, its prevention and causes from the non-missionary sources (Table 4.5). Similarly, in the Lamka town the women have also obtained their information from the non-misionary sources (Table 4.13), very few of the women in both the areas have acquired the information from the missionary sources. Among the female adolescents information pertaining to the menstrual cycle, usage of sanitary napkins, drying of the menstrual cloth as well as cleanliness regime during the cycle have all been disseminated on a large scale by the non-missionary sources (Table 4.22).

(d) Reproductive Health Programme

In regard to the knowledge pertaining to small family norm, immunization during pregnancy, identification of high risk pregnancy etc., the Takvom village women did not receive any information from the missionary source (Table 4.6), however, very few of the Lamka town women received information about the immunization of women during pregnancy from the missionary sources (Table 4.14). Nevertheless, in both the study areas majority of the women derived their information pertaining to the Reproductive Health Programme from the non-missionary sources. Similarly, among the female adolescent the information have also been acquired from the non-missionary source (Table 4.23).

(e) Utilization of Contraceptives

The women in both the study areas did not receive any information about contraceptives from the missionary sources (Table 4.7 and Table 4.15). Moreover, contraceptives such as oral pills, condoms, provision for Vasectomy, Tubectomy, MTP and IUCD were supplied by the non-missionary sources to the women of both Takvom village and Lamka town. Out of the total 65 adolescents interviewed, all of them had knowledge about the different types of contraceptives and their source of information was the non-missionary source (Table 4.24 and Table 4.31). None of them got information from the missionary source.

(f) Awareness Regarding Hygiene

Majority of the Takvom village women keep their home clean, store drinking water properly and have constructed toilet outside their home (Table 4.8) and the source of these informations have been the missionary. Similarly, in the Lamka town, the women have also acquired information in regard to hygiene from the missionary sources (Table 4.16). In both the study areas, the non-missionary sources have also disseminated information pertaining to hygiene, the start for which have been done by the missionaries. In contrast, the Adolescent group felt that the non-missionary sources have spread the information regarding the different aspects of hygiene as compared to the missionary sources (Table 4.25 and Table 4.32).

(g) Awareness Regarding Nutrition

In the Takvom village and the Lamka town, the non-missionary sources have played an active role in spreading awareness in terms of caloric intake of an individual, follow of a food routine as well as consumption of a non-vegetarian diet (Table 4.9 and Table 4.17). Information has also been received from the missionary sources but it is much lesser as compared to the non-missionary sources. Similarly, among the female adolescents, majority of them felt that the non-missionary sources have spread information regarding nutrition (Table 4.26), however, among the male adolescents none of them felt that the missionary have spread information in terms of nutrition they gave the credit to the non-missionary source only (Table 4.33).

(h) Knowledge about Puberty

Female adolescent have acquired their information regarding puberty and the physical changes in boys from the non-missionary sources (Table 4.19). Similarly, among the male adolescent, majority of them received information about puberty and the physical changes in girls from the non-missionary sources

(Table 4.28). Little information about puberty has also been received from the missionary source by both the adolescent group.

(i) Educational Institutions

Majority of the adolescent group interviewed are enrolled in the missionary schools as the medium of teaching is English, quality of teachers is good as well as the teaching technique is better than the non-missionary schools (Table 4.27 and Table 4.34). Moreover they even have classes on value education, career counselling and personality training as well.

Conclusion

The life of tribal women has been deteriorating over the decades. Poverty, lack of basic necessities and exploitation by non-tribals have been the problems faced by all tribes, along with environmental degradation. Destructuion of forests, the lifeline of tribal economy, has hit the tribals areas.

There is an urgent need for gender specific policies to reduce inequalities because the causes of inequalities may be different for men and women. Women should be recognized in their own rights and because of women's crucial importance for health issues they should be included directly and with full responsibility in the planning, decision making and implementation of health-care systems.

To make this possible education is an important factor. Education is intrinsic to development. Empowering people with the basic skills and habits would render them to lead a healthy life. Mother's education enhances the possibility of a child's survival so, in order to raise the health standards, the education standards should also be raised.

Importance of tribal women has been emphasized. Subsequently, State and Central Governments have been launching educational and health awareness programmes for them. With literacy rate moving up, health and hygiene awareness increasing and legislations and norms safeguarding their well-being coming into force, tribal women can look ahead for better times.

The upliftment of tribal women depends much on providing education. Education in the modern world is not only a process of learning and becoming wiser but also a tool at one's command to survive in this age of competition. Those who have not acquired or have been denied this tool, are at a tremendous disadvantage *vis-a-vis* modern living because it is no longer possible in this world today for any society to remain untouched by modern civilization.

One of the significant factors regarding female literacy and educational level among the tribal women is that prior to independence, a number of tribes came under the influence of Christian missionaries and after embracing Christianity took to education.

Earlier people have got used to ill-health and it was seen as a part of their life. The problems in accessibility, quality of services and prices in health care and services are seen as a burden, when weigh against their income. Hence, as long as it does not hamper their day to day routine they would not seek care. More of community empowerment/awareness were needed in order to enable them to demand their own right, development and health needs.

The Paite women of Churachandpur district have also developed a greater level of awareness due to the coming of Christian missionaries into the district and thereby adopting education. They have been, as compared to the earlier times much more aware regarding their health in terms of reproductive health and hygiene.

Initially, for them seeking care for their ill-health was not considered important as long as they are able to continue carrying out household chores or working in the fields. Now there has been a shift in their health seeking pattern. The numbers of women who seek care during pregnancy have gone up to at least 40 per cent as compared to the earlier times (DFWO, Churachandpur). Even their traditional healing process, *i.e. tangal* for vaginal irritation, is no longer used. The women in both the study area have, in more ways than one acknowledged the presence of the missionaries in the district and they felt that the missionaries have definitely paved the way in bringing about awareness among them which in turn have been passed on to their children.

The adolescent groups in Churachandpur district have access to greater facilities in terms of education. This has further expanded their scope of knowledge and their questioning ability. Their awareness regarding the various happenings in and around the country and the world at large has also been enhanced. Comparatively, their educational choices have been more than their parents. At present at least 40 per cent of the adolescents from the Churachandpur district are studying in Delhi and majority of them are doing their graduation and the others pursuing higher studies. This is a remarkable change when 10 years down the line no one ever imagined that they would be studying outside their home town.

Since the town have developed after the arrival of missionaries and education *per se,* the adolescent are less aware about the role played by the missionaries. However, they do believe that the missionaries have started the process of educating the tribal people not only in terms of academics but also personal health and hygiene.

At this stage, in Churachandpur modern medical facilities are available and now easily accessible to the people. It is felt that if the young mothers are made aware of health, personal hygiene, nutrition and utilization of health services, only then there will be a considerable improvement in the health status of women.

The Different Churches in Lamka

1. Evengelical Congregational Church of India (ECCI)
   (a) Evangelical Assembly Church (EAC)
   (b) Evangelical Organization Church (EOC)
   (c) Evangelical Churches Association (ECA)
   (d) Evangelical Synod Church (ESC)
   (e) Evangelical Thangkhal Christian Association (ETCA)
   (f) South East Manipur Christian Association (SEMACA)
2. Manipur Baptist Convention (MBC)
   (a) Chin Baptist Association (CBA)
   (b) Gangte Baptist Association (GBA)
   (c) Kuki Baptist Convention (KBC)
   (d) Vaiphei Baptist Association (VBA)
   (e) Chongthu Baptist Association (CHBA)
3. New Testament Bapitst Churches Association (NTBC)
4. Evangelical Baptist Church (EBC)
5. Fundamental Baptist Church (FBC)
6. Evangelical Free Church of India (EFCI)
7. Zomi Christian Church (ZCC)
8. Presbyterians:
   (a) Tuithaphai Presbytery
   (b) Manipur Gam Presbytery
   (c) Manipur Eastern Presbytery
   (d) Khuga Sadar Presbytery
9. Reformed Presbyterian Church (North East India)
10. Presbyterian Church of India (reformed)
11. Baptist Church of Manipur
12. United Pentecostal Church
13. Assemblies of God
14. Lutheran Church of India

15. Church of God (7th day)
16. Seventh Day Adventist
17. Roman Catholic
18. Salvation Army
19. Church of Christ
20. Meitei Christian Church
21. Assembly of Yahweh
22. House of Yahweh
23. Bet Hashim Midrash
24. Bel-el Church
25. Mount Zion Church of God
26. Spiritual Sabbatarian
27. Orthodox Judaism
28. Israel
29. Family of Elohim
30. Lal Chhungkua
31. Independent Church of God
32. Spiritual Church
33. Revival Church of God
34. Church of Jesus Christ
35. Evangelical Christian Association.

(Hatzaw, 2003, 71)

Glossary

AIDS	Acquired Immune Deficiency Syndrom
DFWO	District Family Welfare Officer
FPP	Family Planning Programme
HIV	Human Immune Virus
IAS	Indian Administrative Service
ICPD	International Conference on Population and Development
IEC	Information, Education and Communication
IPS	Indian Police Service
IUCD	Intra Uterine Control Device
IPPI	Intensified Pulse Polio Immunization
MTP	Medical Termination of Pregnancy
NEFA	North-East Frontier Agency
NGO	Non-Governmental Organization
NPP	National Population Policy
OPD	Out Patient Department
RCH	Reproductive Child Health
RH	Reproductive Health
RTI	Reproductive Tract Infection
SDO	Sub-Divisional Officer
STD	Sexually Transmitted Disease
STI	Sexually Transmitted Infection
TFR	Total Fertility Rate

Questionnaire

Personal Data

Please give the following information:

1. Socio-Demographic Profile:

Name	*Age*	*Sex*	*Marital Status*	*Religion*	*Tribe*	*Edu. Qual.*	*Occ.*	*Family Income*

* Edu.—Educational Qualification.
* Occ.—Occupation.

2. Type of House:
   (a) House Material Used.
   Brick/cement (   ) Wood (   ) Bamboo (   )
   (b) No. of rooms (   )
   (c) Electricity facility available:
   Yes (   ) No (   )

3. Health:
   (a) Did any family member(s) suffer from any illness in the past 3 months?

Family Member	*Illness*	*Duration*	*Care sought*

   (b) Where do you go for your health care?

   (c) To whom do you go and why?

Hygiene, Health and Nutrition

1. Toilet facility.—Yes ( ) No ( )
   Location: Inside house ( ) Outside house ( )
   Type: Flush facilities ( ) Without Flush ( )
2. Water facility. Yes ( ) No ( )
   Localtion: Inside house ( ) Outside house ( )
   Type: Pipe ( ) Tank ( ) Bore water well ( )
   Duration of supply:
3. How many times do you eat in a day?
4. What do you prefer to have for food?
5. What do you usually have for food?
6. Are you aware of the required caloric intake for an individual?
7. How many times in a day/week do you eat non-vegetarian food?

Adolescent Health and Menstrual Hygiene

1. What is your understanding about puberty?

2. Are you aware of the physical changes the boys body undergoes as they reach puberty? Yes (   ) No (   ).
   If yes, mention

   Source of Information

3. Are you aware of the physical changes the girls body undergoes as they reach puberty? Yes (   ) No (   ).
   If yes, mention

   Source of Information

4. Did you know about the menstrual cycle before it happened to you?
   Yes (   ) No (   )
   Source of Information

5. Are you aware about the duration of the menstrual cycle?
   Yes (   ) No (   )
6. Is your menstrual cycle regular?
   Yes (   ) No (   )
7. If irregularity occurs what could be the reason(s)?

8. If you do not menstruate for a month or two, does it mean you are pregnant (   ) anaemic (   ) Other, specify

   Source of Information

9. What do you use during your menstrual cycle to control the blood flow?
   Pad ( ) Cloth ( ) Other, specify

   Source of Information

10. If you use pads for protection how many do you use for one cycle?

11. What are the month's expenses for it?

12. How do you dispose your pads?

13. If you used a cloth do you wash it and re-use it again?
    Yes ( ) No ( )
14. Where do you dry the menses cloth?

15. Do you keep away from religious activities during your menstrual cycle?
    Yes ( ) No ( )
    Why?

Reproductive Health

1. Are you aware of your reproductive organs?
   Yes ( ) No ( )
   Specify

   Source of Information

2. Are you aware of the reproductive ill health problems, such as, vaginal discharge ( ) RTI ( ) STI ( )
   Others, please specify

   Source of Information

3. Have you ever experienced any of the reproductive ill health problems?
   Yes ( ) No ( )
   Please specify

4. How did you recognize it
   Through doctors ( ) Through elder women ( )
   Others, please specify

5. Have you sought any care regarding the problems?

6. If yes, where do you go to seek the care?
   Hospital ( ) PHC ( ) Private Nursing ( )
   Polyclinic ( )
7. What is the source of your information for that care?

8. What are the common symptoms of RTI/STI you are aware of?

9. What are the treatments and preventive methods of RTI/STI you are aware of?

10. Have you heard of AIDS, If yes specify

    Source of Information:

11. Have you heard of the reproductive health programme?
    Yes ( ) No ( )
    If yes, specify

    Source of Information

12. Do you have any knowledge about contraceptive?
    Yes ( ) No ( )
13. Name the contraceptive you are aware of?

    Source of Information

14. Have you ever used any contraceptive?
    Yes ( ) No ( )
15. Are you using any contraceptive at present?
    Yes ( ) No ( )
16. If yes, where do you procure your contraceptive from?
    Chemist ( ) Hospital ( ) other, specify

17. What is your wife/husband perception about using contraceptive?

18. Do you think women should initiate family planning?
    Yes ( ) No ( ) Why?

Family Life Education

1. Do you think family life education should be imparted in school?

2. What issues/components you wish to be covered in the family life education?

3. Have you ever talked to your adolescent child regarding sexuality and reproduction?
   Yes ( ) No ( )
4. In your opinion can media play a role in disseminating the information on sexuality and reproduction?
   Yes ( ) No ( )
   How?

5. Do you think teachers should also disseminate the information?
   Yes ( ) No ( )
   Give reason(s):

6. Is the peer group helpful in disseminating the information?

7. Where did you get the information about sexuality and reproduction:
   parents ( ) teachers ( ) peer group ( )
   media ( )
   If media, specify whether
   print ( ) audio ( ) visual ( )
8. At what age did you acquire the information on sexuality and reproduction?

Missionaries Activities

Hygiene, health and nutrition

- Did the presence of missionaries increase the awareness level in terms of hygiene? Yes ( ) No ( )
- Did the presence of missionaries increase the awareness level in terms of health? Yes ( ) No ( )
- Did the presence of missionaries increase the awareness level in terms of nutrition? Yes ( ) No ( )

  Give reasons for your answer:

I. Infrastructure:

(a) Did the missionary help in the construction of roads?
Yes ( ) No ( )

(b) Did the missionary provide any assistance in making electricty available?
Yes ( ) No ( )

II. Education:

(a) Did the missionary play any role in spreading awareness about education?
Yes ( ) No ( )

(b) Did the missionary open educational institution?
Yes ( ) No ( )

(c) Do you think information about sexuality and reproduction have been more enhanced because of the presence of the missionaries?
Yes ( ) No ( )

(d) Did the missionary put an effort to make the government do the above mentioned job?
Yes ( ) No ( )

(e) Did the missionary seek the assistance of the NGOs to do the above mentioned job?
Yes ( ) No ( )

(f) Did the missionary mobilize the community to do the job with them?
Yes ( ) No ( )

III. Health:

(a) What has been the health status before the arrival of the missionary?

(b) Did the missionary play a role in disseminating information about adolescent health and menstrual hygiene? Yes (   ) No (   )

(c) Did the activities of the missionary help in developing better understanding about youth? Yes (   ) No (   )

(d) Was the knowledge about contraceptive prevalent before the arrival of the missionary? Yes (   ) No (   )
Specify:

(e) Did the missionary set up any hospital/clinic to cater to the need of women? Yes (   ) No (   )

(f) The process of immunization was prevalent before the arrival of the missionary? Yes (   ) No (   )

(g) The morbidity rate among the women decrease with the arrival of the missionary? Yes (   ) No (   )

(h) The health facility for the elderly improve after the missionary came? Yes (   ) No (   )

(i) Did the missionary set up old-age home?
Yes (   ) No (   )

Bibliography

Barpujari, H.K., (1965): *Assam in the the days of Company 1826-1856,* Gauhati.

Basu, A., (1990): 'Anthropological Approach to Tribal Health' in *Tribal Demography* (ed.) by Ashish Bose *et al.* B.R. Publishing, Delhi.

Basu, S.K., (1993): Health Status of Tribal Women in India, *Social Change,* Vol. 23, No. 4.

Bose, Nirmal Kumar, (1971): *Tribal Life in India,* New Delhi, p. 65.

Chatterjeee, K.K., (1993): Health Status of Tribal Women, *Social Change,* December, Vol. 23, No. 40, pp. 16-19.

Downs, Fredericks (1983), *Christianity in Northeast India,* Delhi, p. 185.

Dubey, S.M., (1969): "Education, Social Change and Political Consciousness among the Tribes of North East India", in K. Suresh Singh: *Tribal Situation in India.*

Dubey, S.M., (1969): "Modernization among the Tribes of North-East India", Seminar Paper on Tradition and Modernization, New Delhi.

Haralambos, M. with Heald R.M., (1980): *Sociology: Themes and Perspectives,* Oxford University Press, London, p. 173.

Hatzaw, H.S., (2003): *Christianity in Manipur,* New Lamka, Manipur, pp. 78-80.

Jejeebhoy, J. Shireen (1999): "Reproductive Health Information in India: What Are the Gaps?", *Economic and Political Weekly,* October 16-23.

Jejeebhoy, Shireen J., (1999): "Access to Quality Reproductive Health Care—Preproductive Health Information in India", *Economic and Political Weekly,* October 16-23.

Kishore, J., (2002): *National Health Programmes in India—National Policies and Legislation related to Health,* 4th edition, Century Publication, New Delhi, pp. 15-18.

Ostergaad, Lise, (1992): *Gender and Development,* Routledge, London.

Mukhopadhyay, Lipi, (2002): *Tribal Women in Development,* Publications Division, Ministry of Information and Broadcasting, Government of India, New Delhi, pp. 293-305.

Narain, Raj, (1977): *Family Welfare Programme: Statement of Policy,* New Delhi, Government of India.

Qadeer, Imrana, (2000): "Reproductive Health—Public Health Perspective", *Economic and Political Weekly,* October-December, Vol. 33.

Ray, Ranjana and Banerjee, Jayanta, (1993): Health Status among Tribal Women, *Social Change,* December, Vol. 23, No. 4.

Reddy, P.H., (1994): Population Policy Choices in India, *Social Change,* September-December Vol. 3, No. 4, p. 24.

Reproductive and Child Health (2000): National Institute of Health and Family Welfare, June, New Delhi, pp. 441-443.

Roy, T.K., (1997): Analysis of India's Population Policy: An Experience of Five Decades, *IASSI Quarterly,* 16, Vol. 3, No. 4.

Singh, Karan, (1976): "National Political Policy: Statement," New Delhi, Government of India.

Subba, T.B., Ghosh, G.C., (Ed.) (2003): *The Anthropology of North-East India—A Textbook,* Orient Longman, New Delhi.

Sword, V.K., (1840): *Baptist in Assam—India's Political Consulta-tions,* May 11.

UNESCO: *Dictionary of Social Sciences* (1969), The Free Press.

Upa Luaizakham, (1991): *Nidanglai Hinkhua leh Tuni,* Lamka Printing Press, pp. 23-25.

Index